ORTHOPAEDIC EXAMINATION

Commissioning Editor: Fiona Conn
Development Editor: Clive Hewat
Project Manager: Nancy Arnott
Designer: Erik Bigland

ORTHOPAEDIC EXAMINATION

MADE EASY

JAVAD PARVIZI MD FRCS

Associate Professor of Orthopedic Surgery
Rothman Institute at Thomas Jefferson University
Philadelphia, USA

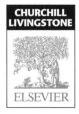

CHURCHILL
LIVINGSTONE

ELSEVIER

EDINBURGH LONDON NEW YORK OXFORD PHILADELPHIA
ST LOUIS SYDNEY TORONTO 2006

CHURCHILL
LIVINGSTONE
ELSEVIER

© 2006, Elsevier Limited. All rights reserved.

The right of Javad Parvizi to be identified as author of this work has been asserted by him in accordance with the Copyright, Designs and Patents Act 1988

No part of this publication may be reproduced, stored in a retrieval system, or transmitted in any form or by any means, electronic, mechanical, photocopying, recording or otherwise, without the prior permission of the Publishers. Permissions may be sought directly from Elsevier's Health Sciences Rights Department, 1600 John F. Kennedy Boulevard, Suite 1800, Philadelphia, PA 19103-2899, USA: phone: (+1) 215 239 3804; fax: (+1) 215 239 3805; or, e-mail: *healthpermissions@elsevier.com.* You may also complete your request on-line via the Elsevier homepage (http://www.elsevier.com), by selecting 'Support and contact' and then 'Copyright and Permission'.

First published 2006

ISBN–10 : 0-443-10001-2
ISBN–13 : 978-0-443-10001-7

British Library Cataloguing in Publication Data
A catalogue record for this book is available from the British Library

Library of Congress Cataloging in Publication Data
A catalog record for this book is available from the Library of Congress

Notice
Knowledge and best practice in this field are constantly changing. As new research and experience broaden our knowledge, changes in practice, treatment and drug therapy may become necessary or appropriate. Readers are advised to check the most current information provided (i) on procedures featured or (ii) by the manufacturer of each product to be administered, to verify the recommended dose or formula, the method and duration of administration, and contraindications. It is the responsibility of the practitioner, relying on their own experience and knowledge of the patient, to make diagnoses, to determine dosages and the best treatment for each individual patient, and to take all appropriate safety precautions. To the fullest extent of the law, neither the Publisher nor the Author assumes any liability for any injury and/or damage to persons or property arising out or related to any use of the material contained in this book.
The Publisher

your source for books,
journals and multimedia
in the health sciences
www.elsevierhealth.com

The
Publisher's
policy is to use
paper manufactured
from sustainable forests

Printed in China

PREFACE

Research has shown that one out of every three patients presenting to a general practitioner complains of symptoms related to the musculoskeletal system. Thus, regardless of what specialty a physician is practicing he or she is likely to encounter patients with musculoskeletal symptoms on a frequent basis. It is therefore imperative that one is proficient in examination of the musculoskeletal system. This book aims to provide the reader with a simple, fast, and effective method of examination of the musculoskeletal system.

Each chapter is structured to provide a brief description of the joint and its components in order to convey to the reader the normal biomechanics of the joint. This in turn allows the reader to formulate a plan for what the expected motion for that joint should be and to interpret the abnormal findings in light of the basic anatomy and biomechanics.

The examination of each joint involves the simple steps of Inspection, Palpation, Range of Motion, and Neurovascular assessment. As the human body is symmetrically bilateral the examiner has the opportunity to compare each component of the examination with the possibly normal contralateral side. Some conditions, however, are bilateral and this should be borne in mind during the examination.

One of the most informative parts of the examination is to observe the patients as they walk into the office or the examination room. This provides the examiner with information regarding body posture, speed of walking, gait abnormalities (such as Trendelenberg gait which is seen with painful hip), ability to carry weight with the upper extremities, and the use of a walking aid. Neurovascular assessment of the extremities is also a crucial part of the musculoskeletal examination. Some vascular and neurological conditions may present with 'muscular' symptoms and be mistaken for musculoskeletal conditions. Some patients with true musculoskeletal pathology may in addition have neurovascular abnormalities which may influence the management of that condition. For example, patients with severe arthritis of the knee and vascular insufficiency will not be good candidates for knee replacement because of potential problems with wound healing. Another common example is the 'co-presentation' of back and hip pain. It is critical that the back and the hip are examined thoroughly in these patients in order to determine the exact etiology for pain, if possible.

Each chapter also presents some of the common tests and signs used to reach a diagnosis. There are examples of some of common conditions and the expected abnormal findings for these conditions are presented.

JP

ACKNOWLEDGMENTS

I would like to thank Leah Bernstein MD and Aidin Eslampour MD for their extensive help with this book particularly in preparation of the figures. I would also like to thank all my surgical colleagues at the Rothman Institute for their encouragement and proof-reading of the chapters for accuracy and relevance.

CONTENTS

History

HISTORY

Accurate history taking and thorough examination of the musculo-skeletal system is an important, yet simple, task. Examination centers mostly on the symptomatic joint but should include the nerves and the muscles that are responsible for motion of the joint and comparison should be made with the contralateral joint, when present.

The complete examination of the musculoskeletal system begins with full history taking.

Like all other systems in the body, accurate history constitutes the most important part of the evaluation. The history begins by determining the demographics for the patient and continues with elucidating the details of the symptoms. Family history, social history, drug history and systematic enquiry are also critical parts of the evaluation.

- Demographics (height, weight, age)
- Details of symptom such as pain:
  - duration
  - site
  - character or nature e.g. shooting pain often is often related to a nerve pain
  - intensity (often expressed as part of Visual Analog Scale: 0= no pain, 10 = worst pain possible)
  - precipitating factors (such as history of trauma)
  - relieving factors
  - exacerbating factors
  - constant or intermittent
  - associated factors such as numbness, stiffness, weakness
  - night pain/rest pain
- Past medical/surgical/anesthesia history (for example previous meniscectomy predisposes the patient to arthritis of the knee; fracture healing is retarded in diabetic patients)
- Drug history and allergies
- Social history: wound and fracture healing is retarded in smokers. The patient's living circumstances are important

- Systematic enquiry
- Family history: some conditions, such as lupus or psoriasis, may present with joint pain.

INSPECTION

The symptomatic joint and the contralateral joint, as well as joints proximal and distal to the affected joint, should be exposed. The joint should be scrutinized for the presence of the following:

- Swelling (diffuse swelling is often a sign of systemic disease or conditions affecting the venous or lymphatic drainage of the limb, whereas localized swelling signifies joint distension from fluid)
- Scars
- Symmetry
- Skin changes (rash, discoloration, abrasion, etc.)
- Shape (deformity, altered posture of the spine)
- Shortening.

PALPATION

The affected joint should at first be gently palpated. Then tenderness in the joint line, tendon or ligament attachment and specific regions around the joint should be evaluated.

- Temperature (warm joint with infection and trauma and cold skin with impaired circulation)
- Swelling (may be palpable)
- Tenderness (specific regions around the joint and attachment of tendons and ligaments should be palpated).

RANGE OF MOVEMENT (ROM)

Assessment of ROM is an essential part of orthopaedic examination. Stiffness is usually associated with arthritis; crepitus with motion is also a sign of arthritis. Fixed deformities are associated with contracture of muscle, tendon or joint capsule. A goniometer may be used to measure ROM of the joints.

NEUROVASCULAR EXAMINATION

A general assessment of the muscle power moving the affected joints, sensation of the skin in the extremity and presence or absence of pulses should be performed. The strength of the muscle contraction is usually expressed using the MRC (Medical Research Council) scale.

MRC SCALE FOR STRENGTH OF MUSCLE CONTRACTION

M5 = normal muscle strength
M4 = some diminished strength (as compared with the contralateral normal side)
M3 = weak but muscle is strong enough to overcome the force of gravity
M2 = muscle can perform work but only if the force of gravity is eliminated
M1 = fasciculations only
M0 = no motor activity at all.

Note that muscle strength may be impaired by pain, denervation, wasting from disuse or systemic diseases.

Sensation of the skin to touch and possibly pin prick should be recorded. The MRC grading for sensation is as follows:

MRC GRADING FOR SENSATION

S4 = normal sensation
S3+ = return of two point discrimination
S3 = return of some superficial cutaneous pain and tactile sensibility but without overreaction
S2 = return of some superficial cutaneous pain and tactile sensibility
S1 = recovery of deep cutaneous pain
S0 = absent sensation in area of affected nerve

SPECIAL TESTS

There are a number of special tests that may need performing to assess the integrity of specific structures, e.g. stress tests for assessment of motion of the joint in abnormal plane; valgus stress applied to the knee (Fig. 1.1) evaluates the integrity of the medial collateral ligament of the knee; anterior drawer test examines the integrity of the anterior cruciate ligament (ACL). Any abnormal (> 5 mm) translation of tibia on the femur upon pulling forward of the tibia on the femur with the knee flexed to 90° signifies loss of ACL constraint (Fig. 1.2).

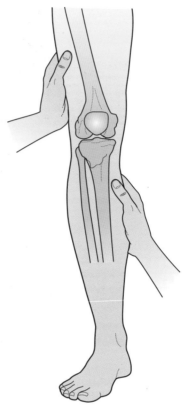

Fig. 1.1
The valgus stress test. One hand is placed on the lateral aspect of the knee while valgus force is applied to the leg. Opening up of the medial knee is indicative of positive test

We present a series of special tests for each joint at the end of each chapter.

EXAMINATION OF RADIOGRAPHS

Close scrutiny of the radiographs is almost always essential for final formulation of a diagnosis for orthopaedic conditions. Some conditions have classic appearances on the radiograph and to an expert eye the condition may be diagnosed based on the radiograph even without examination of the patient. Until such skill is developed analytical review of the radiographs is essential.

The evaluation of radiographs begins with a general scan of the bone, the alignment of the bone and the presence of any gross abnor-

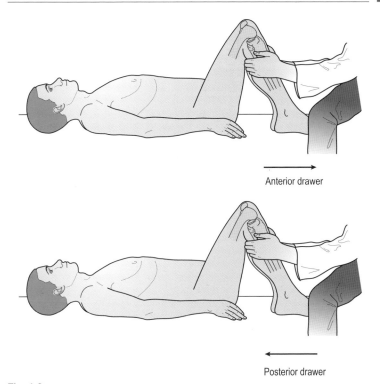

Anterior drawer

Posterior drawer

Fig. 1.2
Anterior drawer test. The knee is held in 90° flexion while the tibia is pulled forward

mality. The quality of the bone (thin cortices in osteoporosis, for example), obvious fractures, or presence of hardware can easily be seen during this general scan. The radiographs are then examined in further detail to detect subtle abnormalities such as calcified menisci, undisplaced fractures, erosions, and other abnormalities.

On occasions special view radiographs may be necessary in order to diagnose a specific condition. For example, posterior dislocation of the shoulder may only be visible in an axillary view of the shoulder.

NOMENCLATURE

Anterior: towards the front of the body.
Arthralgia: pain in the joint.

Arthritis: inflammation of the joint. Implies presence of warmth, swelling, heat, tenderness and possibly erythema.

Baker's cyst: a synovial cyst found in the popliteal space, which may occasionally rupture into the calf and mimic thrombophlebitis.

Body planes: These are three planes – saggital (named after the centaur representing the constellation Sagittarius, as his arrow pointed from the front sections of the body), coronal (in the same plane as a crown being placed on the head) and transverse (slices the body like slices of bread; useful mnemonic, T for toast).

Bouchard's nodes: bony enlargement of the proximal interphalangeal joints found in osteoarthritis.

Bursitis: inflammation of a bursa, which is a synovial lined sac, which may or may not be in communication with a joint cavity.

Crepitation: a palpable or audible grating or crunching sensation produced by motion of a joint or tendon.

Diarthrodial joint: a freely movable joint lined by synovium, such as the knee.

Dislocation: complete loss of congruity between articulating surfaces of a joint.

Fracture: loss of continuity in the cortex of a bone.

- **Avulsion fracture:** a fragment of bone being pulled and avulsed by sudden muscle contraction.
- **Closed fracture:** skin overlying the fracture is not disrupted. Bruising or superficial abrasions may be present.
- **Comminution:** a fracture is comminuted when more than two fragments of bone are present. Degree of comminution is dependant on the amount of energy imparted to the bone during trauma. Butterfly fragment (so called because of its shape) is an example of comminuted fracture.
- **Compression (crush) fracture:** when bone (usually cancellous) receives energy beyond its limit of tolerance and crushes. Usual sites are vertebral bodies and calcaneus (heel) bone.
- **Compound (open) fracture:** wound overlying the fracture allowing communication with the skin and potential for entry of organisms into the fracture.
- **Displacement:** present if the bone ends have shifted relative to one another. The direction of displacement is described in terms of the movement of the distal fragment. Degree of displacement is presented as rough estimates of the percentage of the surfaces in contact.
- **Double fracture:** see segmental fracture.
- **Fatigue fracture:** repeated stresses with excessive frequency applied to a bone that results in fracture. The cortex of the bone may not be completely disrupted.
- **Green stick fracture:** typically occurs in children, but not all fractures in children are of this type. The bone buckles on the

side opposite to the causal force and the thick periosteum may be torn around the fracture.

- **Hairline fracture:** minimal destruction of bone as a result of trauma which is great enough to produce fracture but not severe enough to produce any significant displacement.
- **Impacted fracture:** one fracture fragment driven into another. Fracture is usually fairly stable with no crepitus.
- **Oblique fracture:** the axis of the fracture runs at an angle less than 90° to the long axis of the bone.
- **Pathological fracture:** fracture occurring in an abnormal or diseased bone. Classic examples are fractures in long bones with metastatic disease. Fracture of osteoporotic bone is also, by definition, pathological in nature.
- **Segmental (double) fracture:** bone fractured at two distinct levels leaving a segment of bone inbetween. This must be distinguished from comminuted fracture.
- **Spiral fracture:** the line of fracture curves in a spiral fashion round the bone.
- **Stress fractures:** stress fractures are often hair-line in pattern, and often missed on plain radiographs and not diagnosed with certainty until wisp of periosteal callus formation, or increased density at the fracture site, is seen at a later date (3–6 weeks). Bone scan or MRI is the best modality for diagnosis of stress or fatigue fractures.
- **Transverse fracture:** line of fracture runs perpendicular to the long axis of the bone.

Ganglion: cystic enlargement arising from joint capsules and tendon sheaths, most commonly located on the dorsum of the wrist. In the old days the ganglion used to be ruptured by hitting it hard with a heavy book, such as the Bible.

Heberden's node: bony enlargements of the distal interphalangeal joint of the hand secondary to osteoarthritis.

Kyphosis: rounded thoracic convexity of the spine often seen in older women.

Ligament: connective tissue attaching bone to bone.

Scoliosis: a lateral curvature of the spine.

Sprain: incomplete tear of a ligament or complex of ligaments responsible for the stability of a joint. Sprain may also be applied to incomplete tear of muscle or tendon.

Subluxation: joint surfaces are incongruous but loss of contact is incomplete.

Synovitis: inflammation of the lining tissue of a diarthrodial joint. It results in the palpable swelling of joints found in diseases like rheumatoid arthritis.

Tendon: strong connective tissue attaching muscle to bone.

Tophus: a collection of monosodium urate crystals, which may be palpated beneath the skin in patients with gout.

Valgus: alignment of the limb such that the distal part of the limb points away from the midline of the body.

Varus: alignment of the limb such that the distal part of the limb points towards the midline of the body.

COMMON INJURY LIST

Spine/neck

- Scolosis
- Back pain
- Kyphosis.

Shoulder

- Frozen shoulder
- Rotator cuff tears
- Tendonitis
- Dislocation.

Elbow

- Tennis elbow
- Olecranon bursitis
- Nursemaid's elbow.

Hand/wrist

- Carpal tunnel
- Colles' fracture
- Dupuytren's contracture
- Trigger finger.

Hip/pelvis

- Developmental dysplasia of hip (DDH)
- Slipped femoral epiphysis.

Knee

- Genu varum: 'bow leg'
- Genu valgus: 'knock knee'
- Meniscal tear
- Unhappy triad.

Foot/ankle

- Pes planus: 'flat feet'
- Corns/callosities
- March fracture: the fatigue fracture of the second metatarsal that traditionally occurred in army recruits. Waiter/waitresses are also at risk of this injury.

Life threatening/serious conditions

Septic arthritis

- Musculoskeletal emergency
- Warm, swollen, red joint plus fever
- Prosthetic and diseased joints are predisposed
- Palpation: boggy consistency and decreased ROM.

Compartment syndrome

- Increased tissue pressure within a closed muscle compartment
- Compromise of local circulation and neurological function
- Pain out of proportion to the underlying condition
- On physical examination: severe pain with stretching digits, decreased pulses, weakness, decreased sensation
- Immediate surgery is required to prevent permanent damage.

2

Spine

THE CERVICAL SPINE AND NECK

The cervical spine has three functions: supporting the head, allowing for the head's ROM and housing the spinal cord (Fig. 2.1).

INSPECTION

Normally, the head is held erect and perpendicular to the floor. If it is held stiffly to one side, there may be a pathological condition causing this position.

Inspect to find any abnormalities, like blisters, scars and discoloration. Surgical scars located on the anterior aspect of the neck usually indicate a previous spine or thyroid surgery.

If the base of the skull protrudes anteriorly, suspect cervical or cervicothoracic kyphosis.

PALPATION

Bony palpation

Hyoid bone: located at the level of C3 vertebral body.

Thyroid cartilage: its top portion is called the Adam's apple and is at the level of C4.

Spinous processes: located at the posterior aspect of the neck, in the midline, these are palpable from C2 to T1. C7 and T1 spinous processes are the largest. They are located in line with each other and any shift in their normal alignment may be due to a pathological reason like a facet joint dislocation or fracture.

Facet joints: move your fingers about 2.5 cm lateral to the midline in the back of the neck to palpate facet joints. Assess to see if there is a painful facet or not. The facet joints between C5 and C6 are those which are most often involved in osteoarthritis and may be painful in palpation.

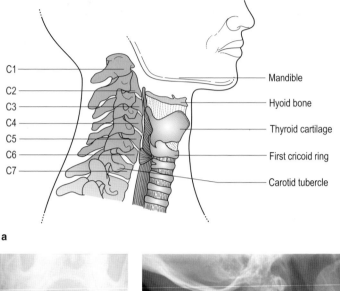

a

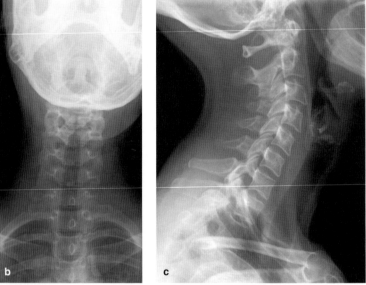

Fig. 2.1
The cervical spine. **a.** Anatomy; **b.** Radiograph, anteroposterior view;
c. Radiograph, lateral view

Soft tissue palpation

Sternocleidomastoid muscle: it extends from the sternoclavicular joint to the mastoid process. Ask the patient to turn the head to the opposite side of the muscle you are palpating. Evaluate the size, shape or tone. Palpate to find any localized swelling that may be due to hematoma in the muscle that may cause torticollis or an abnormally fixed rotation of the cervical spine.

Lymph node chain: located along the medial border of the sternocleidomastoid muscle and anterior border of trapezius muscle. Lymph nodes are not usually palpable. If you find an enlargement in the lymph node chain, it may be due to infection in the upper respiratory tract or, sometimes, to malignancies.

Thyroid gland: situated at the level of C4–5 vertebrae. Normally it feels smooth and indistinct. Palpate to find any enlargement or nodule in the area.

Parathyroid gland: normally is not palpable and the angle of the mandible feels sharp and bony to touch. If enlarged, a baggy, soft gland covers the angle of the mandible.

Supraclavicular fossa: lies superior to clavicle. Palpate to find any unusual swelling or lumps.

ROM

First check the active ROM (Fig. 2.2). If there is any suspicion of unstable cervical spine due to trauma or tumor, do not check the passive ROM:

- Flexion and extension: the patient should be able to touch his chin to his chest (normal range of flexion) and to look directly at the ceiling above him (normal range of extension)
- Rotation (Fig. 2.3): the patient should be able to move the head to both sides so that the chin is in line with the shoulder
- Lateral bending: the patient should be able to bend his head about 45°. It can be limited by enlarged lymph nodes or torticollis.

NEUROLOGICAL EXAMINATION

Muscle testing

Muscle testing of intrinsic muscles

Flexion

- Primary flexors:
  - sternocleidomastoids (spinal accessory nerve, or cranial XI nerve).
- Secondary flexors:
  - scalenus muscles
  - prevertebral muscles.

Extension

- Primary extensors:
  - paravertebral extensor mass (splenius, semispinalis, capitis)
  - trapezius (spinal accessory nerve, or cranial XI nerve).

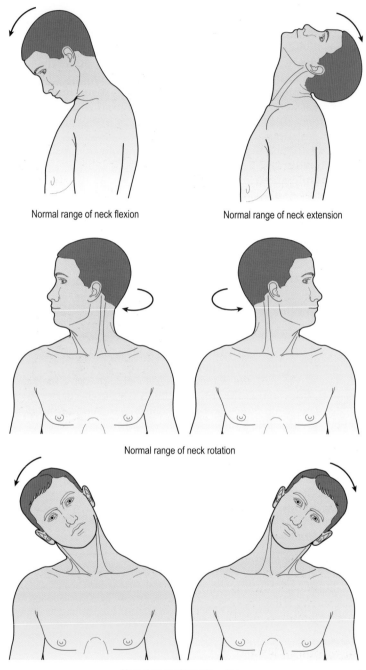

Normal range of neck flexion

Normal range of neck extension

Normal range of neck rotation

Normal range of lateral bending

Fig. 2.2
ROM of the neck

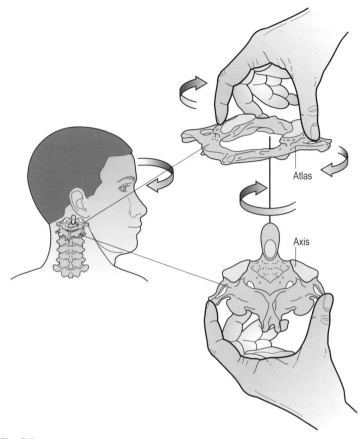

Fig. 2.3
Rotation of the neck

- Secondary extensors:
  - various small intrinsic neck muscles.

Lateral bending

- Primary lateral benders:
  - scalenus anticus, medius, and posticus anterior primary divisions of lower cervical nerves.
- Secondary lateral benders:
  - small intrinsic muscles of the neck.

Neurological levels

The brachial plexus is composed of C5–T1 nerve roots (Fig. 2.4). C5–6 join to make the upper trunk; C8 and T1 join to make the lower trunk

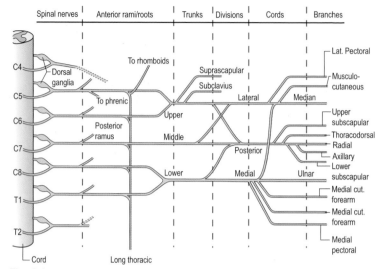

Fig. 2.4
Brachial plexus

and C7 makes the middle trunk. These trunks contribute to make the lateral, middle and posterior cords.

The branches of these cords are:

- Lateral cord:
  - musculocutaneous nerve
  - branch to median nerve.
- Medial cord:
  - ulnar nerve
  - branch to the median nerve.
- Posterior cord
  - axillary nerve
  - radial nerve.

Sensory distribution

C5 nerve root (Fig. 2.5)

- Sensory distribution: lateral arm
- Motor testing: axillary nerve, deltoid muscle
- Musculocutaneous nerve (C5–6), biceps muscle
- Reflex testing: biceps reflex.

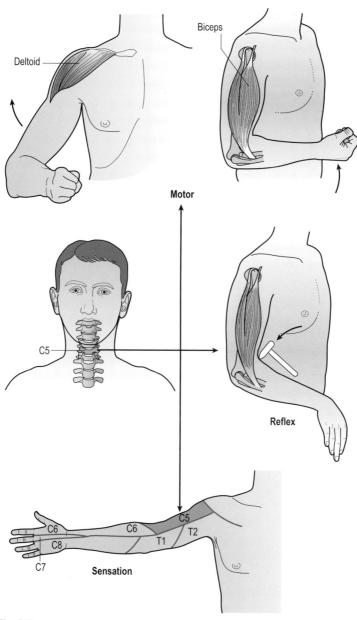

Fig. 2.5
C5 nerve root

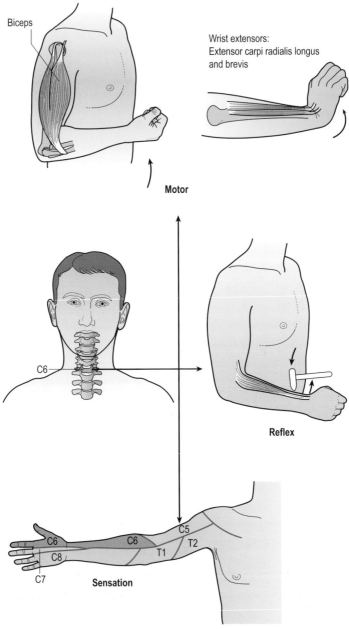

Biceps

Wrist extensors:
Extensor carpi radialis longus
and brevis

Motor

C6

Reflex

C5
C6
C6
T2
C8
T1
C7

Sensation

Fig. 2.6
C6 nerve root

C6 nerve root (Fig. 2.6)

- Sensory distribution: lateral forearm, thumb, index, and half of middle finger (sensory branches of musculocutaneous nerve)
- Motor testing: musculocutaneous nerve (C5–6), biceps muscle
- Wrist extensor group: C6, radial nerve
- Reflex testing: biceps reflex, brachioradialis reflex.

C7 nerve root (Fig. 2.7)

- Sensory distribution: middle finger
- Motor testing: triceps: C7, radial nerve
- Wrist flexor group: C7, median and ulnar nerves
- Reflex testing: triceps reflex.

C8 nerve root (Fig. 2.8)

- Sensory distribution: ring and middle fingers, medial forearm
- Motor testing: finger flexors
  – the flexor digitorum superficialis (proximal interphalangeal (PIP) joint)
  – the flexor digitorum profondis (distal interphalangeal (DIP) joint).

T1 nerve root (Fig. 2.9)

- Sensory distribution: medial arm
- Motor testing: finger abductors
  – the dorsal interossei
  – the abductor digiti minimi (Table 2.1).

Important dermatomes (Table 2.2)

- C2, 3, 4: face
- C4: collar
- T4: nipple.

Table 2.1
Sensory distribution

	Motor levels	Reflexes	Sensory levels
C5	Shoulder abduction	Biceps	Lateral arm
C6	Wrist extension	Brachioradialis	Lateral forearm
C7	Wrist flexion, finger extension	Triceps	Middle finger
C8	Finger flexion	–	Middle forearm
T1	Finger abduction	–	Middle arm

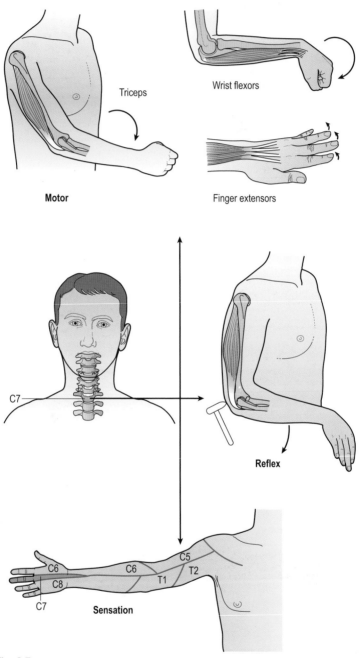

Triceps

Wrist flexors

Motor

Finger extensors

C7

Reflex

C5

C6

C6

C8

T1

T2

C7

Sensation

Fig. 2.7
C7 nerve root

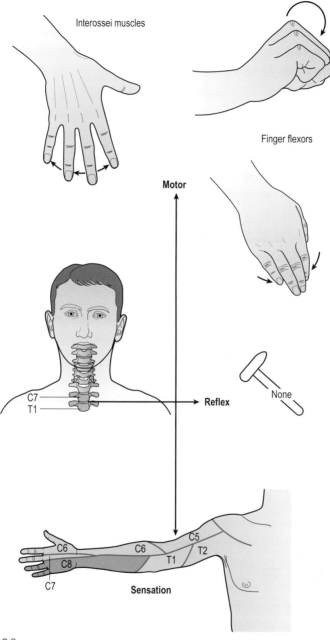

Interossei muscles

Finger flexors

Motor

C7
T1

Reflex

None

C6
C6
C5
C8
T1
T2
C7

Sensation

Fig. 2.8
C8 nerve root

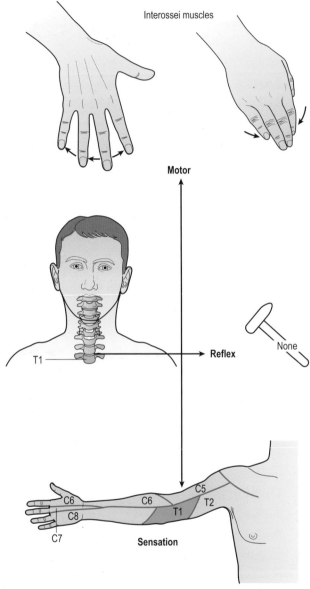

Interossei muscles

Motor

Reflex

None

T1

C5
C6
C6
T2
C8
T1
C7

Sensation

Fig. 2.9
T1 nerve root

Table 2.2
Dermatomes

Disk	Root	Reflex	Muscles	Sensation
C4–C5	C5	Biceps reflex	Deltoid, biceps	Lateral arm, axillary nerve
C5–C6	C6	Brachioradialis, biceps reflexes	Wrist extension, biceps	Lateral forearm, musculocutaneous nerve
C6–C7	C7	Triceps reflex	Wrist flexors, finger extension, triceps	Middle finger
C7–T1	C8, T1	–	Finger flexion, hand intrinsics	Medial forearm, medial anterior brachial cutaneous nerve
T1–T2	T1, T2	–	Hand intrinsics	Medial arm, medial brachial cutaneous nerve

SPECIAL TESTS

Sperling's maneuver: extension and ipsilateral rotation of the neck should produce patient's radicular pain (very specific test).

Lhermitte's sign: so-called Barber Chair phenomenon. Flexion or extension of the neck produces electric shock-like sensations that extend down the spine and shoot into the limbs. When positive, this test signifies spinal cord compression from trauma, multiple sclerosis, cervical cord tumor, cervical spondylosis, or even vitamin B12 deficiency.

Distraction test (Fig. 2.10a): this test evaluates the effect of traction on the relief of pain due to narrowing of the neural foramen. Place the palm of one hand under chin and the other one under occiput and gently lift the head and assess its effect on pain.

Compression test (Fig. 2.10b): press the head down gently while the patient is sitting or lying and assess its effect on the pain.

Valsalva test (Fig. 2.10c): Valsalva maneuver increases the pressure of intrathecal space. Ask patient to hold his breath and bear down as if he were moving his bowels. If there is any space-occupying lesion such as a herniated disk or tumor, this maneuver will result in pain radiation to dermatomes innervated by spinal nerves.

Swallowing test (Fig. 2.10d): if there is any pain or difficulty upon swallowing, it may be due to a bony protuberance or osteophytes, hematoma, infection or tumor in the anterior portion of the cervical spine.

Adson test (Fig. 2.10e): it is used to evaluate the condition of the subclavian artery to see if it is compressed by a cervical rib or other pathological conditions. To perform this test, while feeling the pulses of the radial artery, abduct, extend and externally rotate the arm. Then ask the patient to take a deep breath and to turn his head

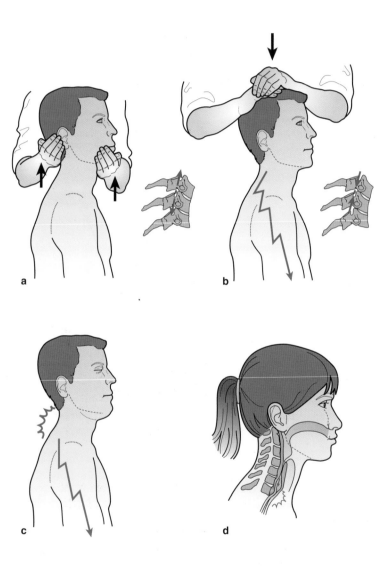

Fig. 2.10
Tests of the cervical spine. **a.** Distraction test; **b.** Compression test; **c.** Valsalva test; **d.** Swallowing test – difficulty in swallowing can be caused by cervical spine pathology

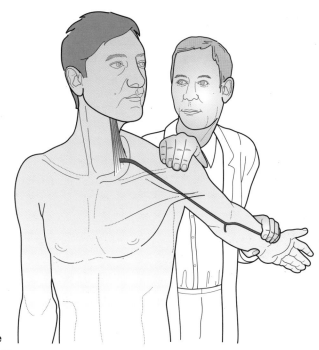

e

Fig. 2.10
e. Adson test

to the opposite side. If there is any compression on the subclavian artery, pulses of the radial artery will be diminished or absent.

LUMBAR SPINE

The lumbar spine (Fig. 2.11) transmits the body weight to the pelvis, provides mobility for the trunk and transports the nerve roots and cauda equina to the lower extremity.

DESCRIPTION OF A FUNCTIONAL SPINAL UNIT

The most common slipped disk occurs at L4–L5 or L5–S1.

Check bowl/bladder incontinence and saddle anesthesia. This is a surgical emergency and the possible sign of cauda equina syndrome (S2–S4).

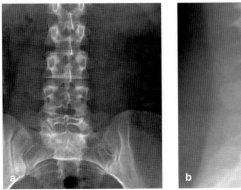

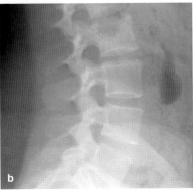

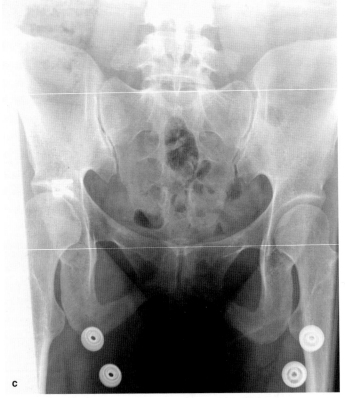

Fig. 2.11
The lumbar spine. **a.** Radiograph – anteroposterior view; **b.** Radiograph – lateral view; **c.** Radiograph – the lumbar spine and pelvis (anteroposterior view)

DESCRIPTION OF COMPONENTS

Bones

Vertebrae

- Spinous processes
- Transverse processes
- Pedicles
- Facet joints: Scotty dog – seen on an oblique plain radiograph (Fig. 2.12). Allows a clear visualization of the pars interarticularis or bone connecting the superior articular process and inferior articular process.

Muscles (origin and insertion)

There are a large number of muscles surrounding the human spine. For details please see anatomy textbooks.

Soft tissues

- Intervetebral disks
- Ligamentum flavum.

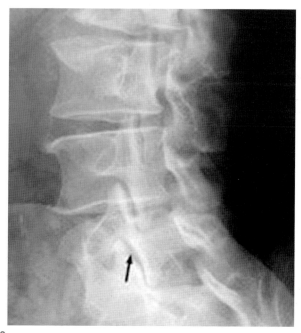

Fig. 2.12
Oblique plain radiograph showing Scotty dog sign

INSPECTION

Check the movements of patient to see whether there is any limitation or rigidity in his movements. When the patient is standing, check for:

- Kyphosis (forward spinal curvature), lordosis (backward spinal curvature) that may be due to weak abdominal musculature and any other abnormal curvatures
- Color changes like café-au-lait spots, birthmarks
- Swelling: lipoma (located in the low back can be a sign of spina bifida)
- Hair patches: an unusual hair patch on the back may be evidence of some bony defects such as spina bifida
- Lacerations
- Bruising
- Asymmetry of the flexion and extension ranges
- Ecchymosis
- Deformities.

PALPATION

The imaginary horizontal line between the tops of the iliac crests passes at the level of L4–5 junction in the midline. The umbilicus lies at the level of L3–4 which is the point where the aorta divides into two branches.
For spasm or pain:

- Spinous processes
- Paraspinal muscles.

ROM

- **Flexion:** ask the patient to bend forward and touch his toes. If he cannot do that, measure the distance between fingertips and floor. Patients with paraspinal muscular spasm will have a problem performing this test. **Extension:** ask the patient to bend backward while you place one hand on the patient's back. Measure and record the range of extension.

NEUROVASCULAR ASSESSMENT

In order to perform a neurological examination of the lumbar spine, perform a complete examination of the lower extremity.

Neurological level T12, L1, 2, 3

- Sensory distribution: general area over the anterior thigh between the inguinal ligament and knee joint
- Motor testing: iliopsoas muscle (nerves from T12, L1, 2, 3) for hip flexion.

Neurological level L2, 3, 4

- Motor testing: quadriceps muscle (L2, 3, 4, femoral nerve) for knee extension
- Hip adductors (L2, 3, 4, obturator nerve).

Neurological level L4

- Sensory distribution: medial side of the leg, below the knee
- Motor testing: tibialis anterior (L4, deep peroneal nerve) for ankle dorsiflexion
- Reflex testing: patellar reflex.

Neurological level L5

Sensory distribution: lateral leg and dorsum of the foot.

- Motor testing:
  - extensor hallucis longus (L5, deep peroneal nerve) for great toe dorsiflexion
  - gluteus medius (L5, superior gluteal nerve) for hip abduction
  - extensor digitorum longus and brevis (L5, deep peroneal nerve).

Neurological level S1

Sensory distribution: lateral malleolus and lateral side and plantar surface of the foot.

- Motor testing:
  - peroneus longus and brevis (S1, superficial peroneal nerve) for ankle eversion
  - gastrocnemius–soleus (S1, 2, tibial nerve) for ankle plantarflexion
  - gluteus maximus (S1, inferior gluteal nerve) for hip extension
- Reflex testing: Achilles' tendon reflex.

Neurological level S2, 3, 4

Sensory distribution: dermatomes around the anus.

- Motor testing:
  - anal wink
  - bladder.

Superficial reflexes

Superficial abdominal reflexes

Ask the patient to lie supine and stroke each quadrant of the abdomen with a sharp end of a pen or neurological hammer. Normally, the umbilicus will move toward that quadrant. The lack of an abdominal reflex indicates an upper motor neuron lesion. The upper quadrant is innervated by T7 to T10 segments of spine and lower quadrant by T11 to L1 segments of spine.

Superficial cremasteric reflex

Stroke the inner side of the thigh with a sharp point of a pen or neurological hammer. In males, normally, the scrotal sac will move upward in the same side. This reflex assesses T12 segment of spine.

Superficial anal reflex

Touch the perianal skin. The external anal sphincter should contract in response. It assesses S2, 3, 4 segments.

Pathological reflexes

These reflexes are mediated by the cerebral cortex and are not present normally in an adult. Their presence indicates an upper motor neuron lesion.

Babinski test

Touch the outer portion of the plantar surface of the foot. Normally, this maneuver results in plantar flexion of foot. An extended great toe, and plantar flexion and splay of other toes, is a positive test and a sign for upper motor lesion. This test can be positive in old people who do not have any pathological condition.

Oppenheim test

Run your finger along the anterior crest of tibia. Normally, there is no reaction; if you do find a response it is also, as with a positive Babinski test, a sign of upper motor neuron lesion.

- Toe walking: S1 provided by gastrocnemius and anterior tibialis. About 50% loss is necessary before a patient is unable to toe walk
- Heel walking: L4, 5 provided by tibialis anterior. Again, about 50% loss is indicated if a patient cannot walk on their heels.

Important dermatomes:

- L4: knee, anterior and medial calf
- L5: lateral calf, dorsum of foot
- S1: posterior calf, lateral foot, perineum.

Motor assessment

- Cervical ROM: flex and extend neck and bend laterally left and right
- Cervical rotation: touch chin to shoulder on left and right
- Lumbar flexio: Schober maneuver – the distance between tip of fingers and floor on forward bending is measured. Loss of flexion occurs with diseases like ankylosing spondylitis.

COMMON TESTS

Straight leg-raising test

Ask the patient to lie supine and lift his leg upward with an extended knee. Normally, you can lift the leg without any complaint of pain from the patient for approximately 80°. If there is any compression on the sciatic nerve, the patient will feel a radiating pain from his back to below the knee. If there is pain at only the posterior aspect of the thigh, it can be due to hamstring muscles.

Cross leg (well leg) straight-raising test

Ask the patient to lie supine and lift his uninvolved leg upward with an extended knee. If there is compression on the sciatic nerve, this maneuver may result in a radiating pain in the posterior aspect of the involved leg to the foot.

Reverse leg-raising test

Ask the patient to lie prone and extend his involved leg with an extended knee. If there is compression on the femoral nerve, this maneuver may result in a radiating pain in the anterior aspect of the involved leg to the foot.

Hoover test

This is used to determine whether a patient who complains of an inability to raise his leg is malingering or not. Ask the patient to lie supine and raise his uninvolved leg while you gently put your hand under the involved foot's calcaneous. If the patient is malingering, you will feel pressure on your hand while the patient tries to raise his uninvolved leg from table.

Milgram test

Ask the patient to lie supine and raise his legs approximately 5 cm from the table. This maneuver stretches the iliopsoas and anterior abdominal muscles and increases the intrathecal pressure. If the patient can hold this position for 30 seconds without any pain in his legs, intrathecal pathology may be ruled out.

3

Shoulder

DESCRIPTION OF THE JOINT

The shoulder joint is a ball and socket joint where the humeral head articulates with the glenoid fossa (Fig. 3.1). It comprises three joints and one articulation: acromioclavicular (AC), sternoclavicular (SC) and glenohumeral (GH) joints and scapulothoracic (ST) articulation. Rotator cuff muscles and tendons support and strengthen the shoulder joint.

The AC joint, like the SC, is a small synovial joint that has limited ROM but withstands significant loads that leads to osteoarthritis of these joints. AC joint degeneration results in painful pathology of the shoulder. AC joint decompression is frequently performed to relieve pain.

The GH joint is a shallow ball and socket articulation that affords tremendous motion. The latter comes at the cost of instability: the shoulder joint is the most commonly dislocated joint in the human body.

Differential diagnosis of shoulder pain focuses on a rotation cuff injury. SITS muscles (rotator cuff muscles: supraspinatus, infraspinatus, teres minor and supscapularis; Fig. 3.2) are prone to overuse because they are modulation muscles more than strength muscles. Supraspinatus is the most common cuff muscle injured. Chronic strain is seen in people who work with their hands above their head e.g. when wallpapering. Patients report pain when reaching for a seat belt or when putting an arm in a coat.

Shoulder joint is the smallest area of articulation compared to available joint space of any joint in the body. Therefore, it is the joint most prone to dislocation. Some factors aiding in stability include muscular constraint, glenoid labrum (deepening the socket), capsule, and ligaments.

DESCRIPTION OF COMPONENTS

Bones (Fig. 3.1)

- Scapula
- Humerus
- Acromion
- Clavicle.

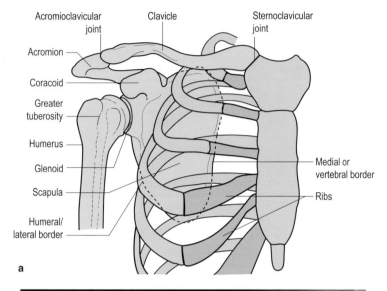

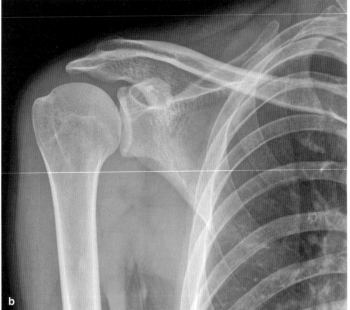

Fig. 3.1
The shoulder joint. a. Anatomy; b. Radiograph (anteroposterior view)

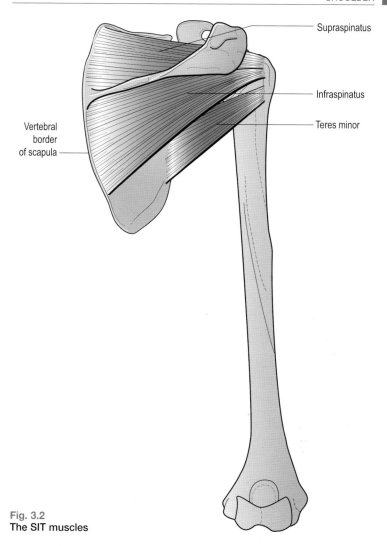

Supraspinatus

Infraspinatus

Teres minor

Vertebral
border
of scapula

Fig. 3.2
The SIT muscles

Muscles

SITS = rotator cuff muscles (supraspinatus, infraspinatus, teres minor and supscapularis).

INSPECTION

The opportunity should be taken to observe the patient while they are walking into the examination room. The posture of the arm, the willingness of the patient to use the arm, symmetry of the shoulders during walking, and the patient's facial expression are all important indicators.

Remove the patient's shirt and observe the shoulder from the front and the back. The shoulder height, evidence of muscle wasting, abnormalities involving the bony contours, swelling, scars, and skin discoloration should be noted. From behind, the scapula should be equidistant from the midline (vertebral column) and flat against the chest wall. High scapula (Sprengel's deformity), winging, and wasting of some of the major muscles (Table 3.1) of the shoulder are only apparent from behind.

The easiest way to determine whether there is any abnormality or not is to compare right and left sides with each other.

The upper extremity swings in tandem with the opposite lower extremity in a normal gait.

Looking at the back, assess:

- Symmetry for discrepancies in scapular height or muscle bulk
- Color changes

Table 3.1
Shoulder muscles

Muscles	Origin	Insertion
Supraspinatus	Supraspinatus fossa	Greater tuberosity of humerus
Infraspinatus	Infraspinatus fossa	Greater tuberosity of humerus
Teres minor	Dorsal surface of axillary border of scapula	Greater tuberosity of humerus
Subscapularis	Internal two-thirds of border of subscapular fossa	Lesser tuberosity
Deltoid	Lateral third of clavicle, acromion process, spine of scapula	Deltoid prominence of humerus
Latissimus dorsi	Spinous process of six inferior dorsal vertebrae, iliac crest, 3–4 lower ribs	Bicipital groove of humerus
Pectoralis major	Medial half of clavicle, sternum, 6–7 ribs	Bicipital groove of humerus
Pectoralis minor	3rd, 4th, and 5th ribs	Coracoid process of scapula

- Lacerations
- Bruising
- Asymmetry of the flexion and extension ranges
- Eccymosis
- Deformities.

Erb's palsy: internally rotated and adducted arm like a waiter asking for tip.

Shoulder dislocation: prominent acromion with the arm slightly held away from the trunk.

Winging scapula: because of weakness or atrophy of serratus anterior or trapezius muscles. Seen by pushing against wall or elevating the arm.

Sprengel's shoulder: high riding scapula because of partially descending scapula.

PALPATION

Bony palpation

This should be performed with the patient relaxed (sitting or lying down). Start palpation from suprasternal notch, sternoclavicular joint and move along the length of clavicle. The acromioclavicular joint is along the lateral border of the clavicle. Motion of the shoulder (especially extension) allows better localization of the AC joint as it moves with the shoulder. Lateral to the AC joint is the flat and broadened acromion process. The next bony landmark is the greater tuberosity of the shoulder. The coracoid process can be palpated just inferior to the AC joint in the deltopectoral triangle. In some patients the bicipital groove can also be palpated just lateral to the lesser tuberosity with the arm in neutral rotation.

The scapula along its medial (vertebral) and lateral (humeral) border as well as its spine should be fully palpable. Motion of the scapula with movement of the arm should also be assessed.

Soft tissue palpation

There are four clinical zones: 1) rotator cuff, 2) subacromial and subdeltoid bursa, 3) axilla, and 4) prominent muscles of shoulder girdle.

Rotator cuff

The rotator cuff is composed of four muscles, in order from anterior to posterior: subscapularis, supraspinatus, infraspinatus, teres minor. The last three can be palpated in a passively extended shoulder. Assess for any tenderness that may indicate rotator cuff syndrome.

Subacromial and subdeltoid bursa

Palpable just below the edge of the acromion in a slightly abducted and extended arm. Assess any tenderness, thickening and crepitation that may indicate bursitis.

Axilla

The armpit is a quadrilateral structure composed of pectoralis major, latisimus dorsi, ribs 2–6 and overlying serratus anterior muscle medially, and bicipital groove of humerus laterally. For palpation first abduct the arm slightly and insert your index and middle fingers into the axilla, then adduct the axilla to relax the skin and make it easier to penetrate higher. Look for any lymph node that is enlarged or tender. The brachial artery pulse can be felt if gentle pressure is applied over the shaft of humerus.

Prominent muscles of shoulder girdle

Examine sternocleidomastoid, pectoralis major, biceps, deltoid, trapezius, rhomboid minor and major, latissimus dorsi and serratus anterior muscles.

Assess for tenderness:

- Bicipital groove
- Subdeltoid area
- Trapezius.

VASCULAR ASSESSMENT

Palpate pulses proximal and distal to joint.

MOTOR ASSESSMENT

Evaluate active ROM first. If there is any asymmetry in active motion or the patient is unable to perform any motion fully, passive testing should be conducted (Fig. 3.3).

Normal active ROM

180° of forward flexion, 60° extension

A limited ROM in flexion and extension movement may indicate bursitis, bicipital tendonitis, arthritis, or adhesive capsulitis (frozen shoulder).

90°internal and external rotation

Internal rotation is best assessed by asking the patient to place their hand on their back and move it up towards the head along the spine. Normally, the patient should be able to reach T2.

Limitation in internal or external rotation may indicate shoulder subluxation, rotator cuff pathology, arthritis, or adhesive capsulitis.

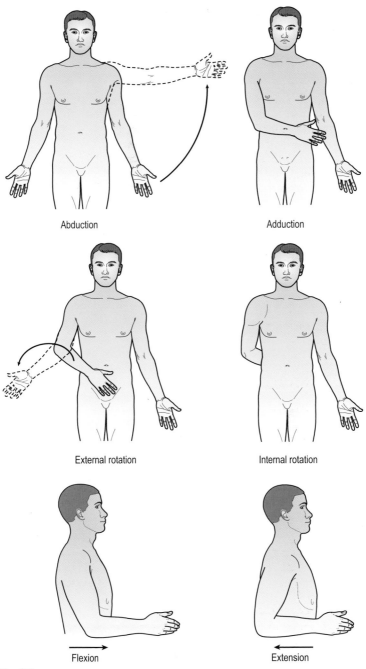

Abduction

Adduction

External rotation

Internal rotation

Flexion

Extension

Fig. 3.3
Shoulder motion

180° abduction, 30° adduction

A limited ROM in abduction and adduction movement may indicate bursitis, rotator cuff syndrome, arthritis, or adhesive capsulitis.

NEUROLOGICAL ASSESSMENT

For assessment of neurological function, muscle strength is evaluated in accordance with a muscle strength chart.

Flexion

Primary flexor muscles

1. Anterior portion of deltoid
   Axillary nerve, C5
2. Coracobrachialis
   Musculocutaneous nerve, C5–C6.

Secondary flexors

1. Pectoralis major (clavicular head)
2. Biceps
3. Anterior portion of deltoid.

Extension

Primary extensor muscles

1. Latissimus dorsi
   Thoracodorsal nerve, C6, C7, C8
2. Teres major
   Lower subscapular nerve, C5, C6
3. Posterior portion of the deltoid
   Axillary nerve, C5, C6.

Secondary extensor muscles

1. Teres minor
2. Triceps (long head).

Abductors

Primary abductor muscles

1. Middle portion of the deltoid muscle
   Axillary nerve, C5–C6
2. Supraspinatus
   Subscapular nerve, C5–C6.

Secondary abductor muscles

1. Anterior and posterior portions of the deltoid muscle
2. Serratus anterior muscle, by direct action on the scapula
   Note: Supraspinatus initiates first 15–20° of abduction.
   Deltoid continues abduction. Abduction is due to combination
   of movements in the glenohumeral and scapulothoracic joints.

Adductors

Primary adductor muscles

1. Pectoralis major
   Medial and lateral anterior thoracic nerve, C5, C6, C7, C8, T1
2. Latissimus dorsi
   Thoracodorsal nerve, C6, C7, C8.

Secondary adductors

1. Teres major
2. Anterior portion of the deltoid muscle.

External rotators

Primary external rotators

1. Infraspinatus
   Suprascapular nerve, C5,C6
2. Teres minor
   Branch of the axillary nerve, C5.

Secondary external rotators
Posterior portion of deltoid.

Internal rotators

Primary internal rotators

1. Subscapular
   Upper and lower subscapular nerve, C5,C6
2. Pectoralis major
   Medial and lateral anterior thoracic nerves, C5, C6, C7, C8, T1
3. Latissimus dorsi
   Thoracodorsal nerve, C6, C7, C8
4. Teres major
   Lower subscapular nerve, C5, C6.

Secondary internal rotators
Anterior portion of the deltoid.

Scapular elevation

Primary elevators

1. Trapezius
   Spinal accessory nerve, or cranial nerve XI
2. Levator scapula
   C3, C4 and frequently branches from the dorsal scapula nerve, C5.

Secondary elevators

1. Rhomboid major
2. Rhomboid minor.

Scapular retraction

Primary retractors

1. Rhomboid major
   Dorsal scapular nerve, C5
2. Rhomboid minor
   Dorsal scapular nerve, C5.

Secondary retractors
Trapezius.

Scapular protraction

Primary scapular protractor

1. Serratus anterior
   Long thoracic nerve, C5, C6, C7.

Sensation testing

- The lateral arm: C5 nerve root
- The medial arm: T1 nerve root
- The axilla: T2 nerve root
- From axilla to nipple: T3 nerve root
- The nipple: T4 nerve root.

SPECIAL TESTS

Apley's scratch test (Fig. 3.4a)

Provides a quick assessment of the combined movement of the shoulder. Ask the patient to bring one hand behind the head and reach the superior border of the scapula on the opposite side (this tests external rotation and abduction). The patient is asked to touch the back with the opposite hand and slide the hand superiorly (this tests the internal rotation and adduction). The movement can then be reversed.

Scapular winging (Fig. 3.4b)

The patient is asked to push against the wall. Scapula becomes prominent. Medial winging of the scapula is the result of injury to the long thoracic nerve (C5, C6, C7) that can occur for example during lymph node resection in the axilla. Lateral winging is the result of trapezius weakness (accessory spinal nerve).

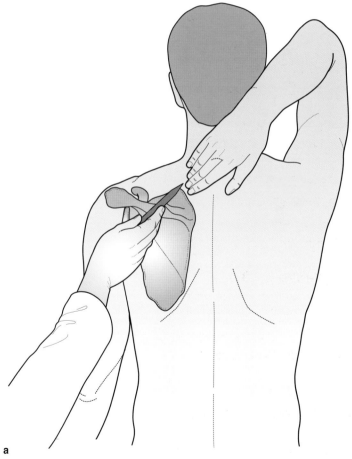

a

Fig. 3.4
Tests of the shoulder joint. **a.** Apley's scratch test

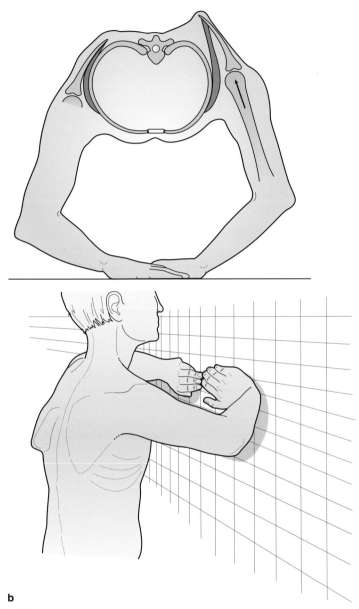

b

Fig. 3.4
b. Scapular winging

Sergeant's badge sensory test (Fig. 3.4c)

This is a rapid, albeit somewhat inaccurate, test for integrity of the axillary nerve. The C5 dermatome over the lateral upper arm (badge area) is tested. The axillary nerve may be injured during shoulder dislocation or following surgery. The best test is to ask the patient to lift the arm and perform isometric deltoid contraction against resistance.

Apprehension test (Fig. 3.4d)

Over 95 % of shoulder dislocations occur anteriorly. Posterior dislocation can occur during seizure or electrocution. Apprehension test is usually positive in patients with recent anterior dislocation or in

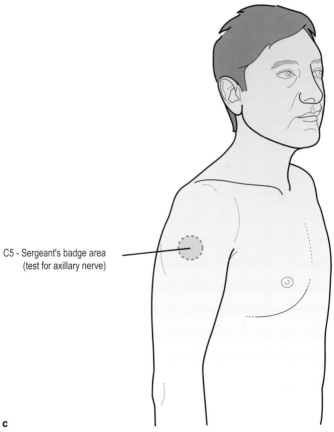

C5 - Sergeant's badge area
(test for axillary nerve)

c

Fig. 3.4 *continued*
c. Sergeant's badge sensory test

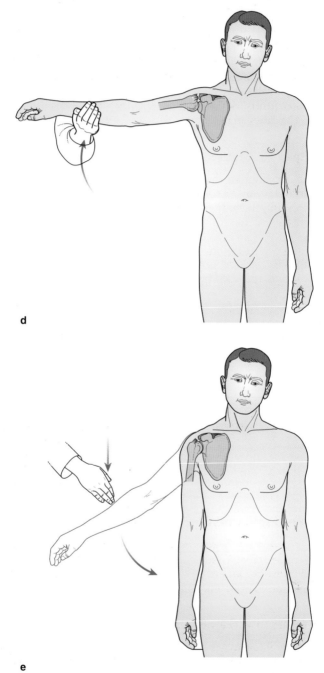

d

e

Fig. 3.4 *continued*
d. Apprehension test; **e.** Drop-arm test

those with continuing anterior subluxation. Lay the patient supine and take their forearm in one hand and support the arm posteriorly, then externally rotate the arm. The test is positive when the patient shows signs of apprehension or resists external rotation in fear of dislocation. Note the degree of external rotation at which the patient exhibits apprehension. The proximal part of the humerus can now be pushed posteriorly by one hand. This may allow further external rotation. The latter maneuver is called the Jobe relocation test.

Tests for impingement syndrome

Narrowing of the subacromial space is caused by osteophytes (AC joint arthritis) or soft tissue swelling (bursitis). This insufficient space creates painful pinching of the rotator cuff between the acromial roof above and the rotator cuff.

- Glenohumoral joint from 0–60°
- Outside 60–120° – pain = 'painful arc'. Impingement
- 120° scapular thoracic movement lifts arm
- ROM signs:
  - Drop-arm sign: hold arm up above head and drop = active abduction to 90°. Pain = increased suspicion for impingement
  - Hawkin's sign: internal rotation and elevation. Evaluate for impingement pain
  - Neer's sign: 90–180° pain = impingement pain.

Drop-arm test (Fig. 3.4e)

The test is performed to evaluate the integrity of the rotator cuff or impingement (see above). Bring the arm to 90° abduction with the elbow fully extended. Ask the patient to lower the arm gently. The result is positive (i.e. there is rotator cuff pathology) if the patient is unable to lower the arm gently and the arm drops to the side with pain.

Hawkin's supraspinatus test (Fig. 3.4f)

With the elbow fully flexed, bring the arm to 90° of abduction, then forcibly internally rotate the arm. This maneuver brings the supraspinatus tendon against the anterior portion of the coracoacromial ligament. Pain is indicative of supraspinatus impingement.

Lift-off test (the Gerber test) (Fig. 3.4g)

This tests the integrity of the subscapular muscle. Ask the patient to place the dorsum of the hand against the back (lumbar spine), and then ask the patient to lift the hand off the back. Inability to perform this test is indicative of supscapular muscle pathology.

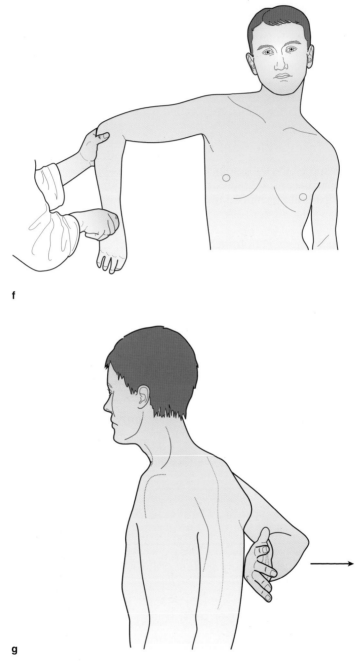

f

g

Fig. 3.4   *continued*
f. Hawkin's supraspinatus test; **g.** Lift-off test

Yergason test (Fig. 3.4h)

While holding the patient's flexed elbow and wrist, externally rotate the arm and pull downward while the patient simultaneously resists. If the biceps tendon is unstable in the bicipital groove, the patient will experience pain.

Speed test of the biceps

This test is to confirm partial rupture of tendonitis of the biceps. The patient sits with the elbow fully extended and arm flexed to 90°. Resisting further flexion of the arm with the forearm in supination will elicit pain in the bicipital groove in a patient with bicipital tendon pathology.

Thoracic outlet syndrome

Thoracic outlet syndrome presents with symptoms or signs of neuro-vascular compression (numbness, tingling, pain, loss of pulse, etc.). The tests attempt to narrow the thoracic outlet.

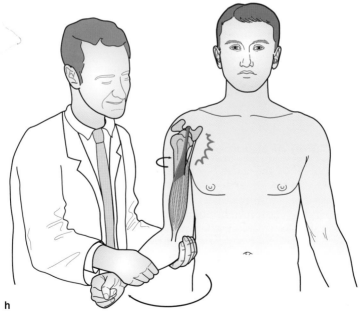

h

Fig. 3.4 *continued*
h. Yergason test

Adson's test

With the patient sitting and your finger on the radial pulse, bring the arm to the side, ask the patient to rotate the chin to face the test shoulder and then extend the neck as far as possible, to take a deep breath and hold it (Valsalva maneuver). Externally rotate and extend the shoulder. This maneuver stretches the scalene anterior muscle. Positive test is when the radial pulse disappears.

Wright's test

With the patient sitting, the outstretched arm is brought to the side while palpating the radial pulse. Ask the patient to turn the head away from the test shoulder and elevate the chin. Now ask the patient to exercise the Valsalva maneuver. The test is positive if symptoms are aggravated or if the pulse disappears.

Roos test

The patient stands, abducts both shoulders to 90°, flexes both elbows to 90°, and externally rotates the arms. The patient is then asked to open and close the fists for three minutes. Precipitation of symptoms such as numbness, weakness, or ischemic pain in the arms and hands is indicative of thoracic outlet syndrome.

COMMON CONDITIONS

Frozen shoulder

Frozen shoulder is a clinical syndrome that is produced by a variety of conditions. Symptoms are limited motion, particularly rotation. Some of the causes include rotator cuff pathology, prolonged period of immobilization, and calcific tendinopathy. The mainstay of treatment is pain relief. Occasionally manipulation under anesthesia may be required.

Dislocation of shoulder

The shoulder is the most commonly dislocated joint in the body. Over 90% of dislocations are anterior. Acute injury (such as a fall onto an outstretched arm) is usually the cause. In younger patients dislocation may become recurrent. Surgical repair of the soft tissues (capsule), and labral lesions (such as Bankart's) may be necessary to prevent recurrence. Beware of habitual shoulder dislocation in patients with psychosis, drug-seeking behavior, or those with sever joint laxity.

Rotator cuff tear

Rotator cuff (RC) tear is a very common condition. It usually occurs as a result of acute injury (such as traction on the arm). Degenerative tear of the RC can also occur. Supraspinatus is the most commonly affected muscle. Symptoms of RC tear includes painful arc of motion, inability to raise the arm above the head, and weakness of rotation.

Impingement syndrome

This painful condition of the shoulder results from formation of osteophytes or soft tissue swelling in the subacromial space.

Arthritis of AC joint

Arthritis is not uncommon in the AC joint. The problem presents with a painful shoulder. On examination, tenderness in the AC joint with or without osteophyte formation can be confirmed. Treatment is usually conservative but occasionally decompression of the joint may be required.

Acute injury to the shoulder can also result in separation of the AC joint. This is also usually treated conservatively.

Fracture of humerus

Fracture of the proximal humerus is common. The fracture is usually below the anatomical neck in the so-called surgical neck area. It is common in elderly women with osteopenia. Treatment depends on the degree of displacement and the number of fracture fragments. Separation of greater than 1 cm or more than 45° determines the 'parts' for fracture. Four-part fracture involves the greater tuberosity, lesser tuberosity, humeral head and the humeral shaft.

Clavicular fracture

Fracture results from a fall. The condition is common in children. Unless the fracture is open or the skin is severely tented the fracture can be treated in a sling and heals uneventfully. Callus formation can occasionally be exuberant and visible through the skin.

4

Elbow

DESCRIPTION OF THE JOINT

The elbow (Fig. 4.1) is a hinge joint that has three major articulations:

- Ulnohumoral
- Humororadial
- Ulnoradial.

A high degree of congruency between the bony elements and the strong ligaments confer good stability to the elbow. ROM of this upper extremity hinge joint is restricted to 135° flexion and full extension is to 0°. Some people have hyperextension of up to 15°.

With the elbow fully extended and the arm by the side, there is a natural outward angulation at the elbow called the carrying angle, which is 7° valgus to prevent the hand from hitting the lower extremity. The angle is higher (10°) for women, as they have wider hips.

Triceps is the major extensor of the elbow joint, although gravity also extends the elbow. Biceps and brachioradialis are major flexors.

Pronation is controlled by pronator teres and pronator quadratus. The biceps and the supinator control supination (place the hand to face the 'sky' – 'S' for supination). The normal rotation of the hand is 90° pronation and 90° supination. The axis of pronation and supination passes through the radial head.

Functional ROM (necessary to perform activities of daily living) is 100° arc of motion. A person could lose up to 30° extension and flex up to 130° with no appreciable sign of loss of function. Functional range of pronation and supination is 50° each.

DESCRIPTION OF COMPONENTS

Bones

Proximal bone – humerus.
Distal bones – medially: ulna; laterally: radius.

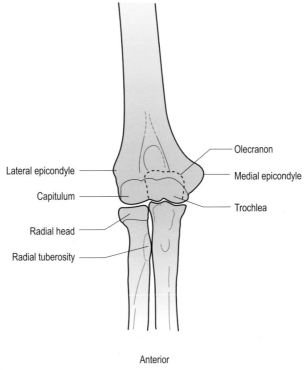

Olecranon

Lateral epicondyle

Medial epicondyle

Capitulum

Trochlea

Radial head

Radial tuberosity

Anterior

a

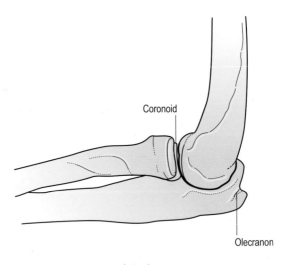

Coronoid

Olecranon

b   Lateral

Fig. 4.1
The elbow joint. a. Anteroposterior view; b. Lateral view

Muscles (Table 4.1)

Common tendons: all extensors or flexors become one tendon and insert at the lateral and medial epicondyle, respectively.

Soft tissues

- Radial collateral ligament
- Ulnar collateral ligament
- Annular ligament of the radius
- Biceps tendon
- Joint capsule
- Oblique cord.

INSPECTION

Look for swelling, muscle wasting, scars, edema, ecchymosis, lacerations, deformities and skin changes. Inspect for nodules (i.e. seen on extensor surfaces in gout and rheumatoid arthritis).

A painful elbow is held in a semi-flexed position as the capsule is least stretched in this position. Ask the patient to extend the elbows and note the carrying angle:

Cubitus valgus: if carrying angle is more than normal (males > 11°, and females >13°).

Cubitus varus (gunstock deformity): if carrying angle is less than normal.

Table 4.1
Muscles of the elbow

Muscles	Origin	Insertion
Biceps	Coracoid process, glenoid cavity	Radial tuberosity
Triceps	Scapula, posterior shaft of humerus	Olecranon
Brachioradialis Brachialis	Distal humerus Distal humerus	Styloid process Proximal ulna
Pronator teres	Medial humeral epicondyle, ulnar head	Anterior radial border
Pronator quadratus	Distal ulna	Distal radius
Supinator	Proximal radius	Ulnar tuberosity

PALPATION

Bony landmarks

- **Laterally:** lateral epicondyle and radial head.
- **Medially:** medial epicondyle: assess for tenderness at medial and lateral epicondyles (i.e. soft tissue injury).
- Olecranon process of ulna.
- Olecranon fossa.

Soft tissue palpation

Medial aspect

- Ulnar nerve: ulnar nerve is situated in the sulcus between medial epicondyle and olecranon. Gently check to assess for tenderness or thickening. Any scar tissue may cause nerve compression and tingling sensation in the patient's ring and little fingers
- Wrist flexor–pronator muscle group
- Medial collateral ligament
- Supracondylar lymph nodes.

Posterior aspect

- Olecranon bursa
- Triceps muscle.

Lateral aspect

- Wrist extensors
- Brachioradialis
- Lateral collateral ligament
- Annular ligament.

Anterior aspect

Cubital tunnel: a triangular space, bordered by brachioradialis muscle laterally, pronator teres muscle medially and an imaginary line drawn between the two epicondyles of the humerus. Structures passing through it from its lateral to medial are:

- Biceps tendon
- Brachial artery
- Median nerve
- Musculocutaneous nerve.

NEUROLOGICAL ASSESSMENT

- Median nerve lies medial to the biceps tendon and superficial to the brachialis muscle
- Radial nerve lies lateral to the biceps tendon

- Ulnar nerve lies at the elbow directly behind the medical epicondyle.

Muscle testing

Flexion
Normal = 145°, functional 30 –130°.

Primary flexors

1. Brachialis
   Musculocutanous nerve, C5, C6.
2. Biceps, in a supinated forearm
   Musculocutanous nerve, C5, C6.

Secondary flexors

1. Brachioradialis
2. Supinator.

Extension
Normal = 0° males, 15° in females.

Primary extensors

1. Triceps
   Radial nerve, C7.

Secondary extensor
Anconeus. Hyperextension is seen in patients with hyperlaxity conditions (such as Ehler–Danlos). Loss of extension or flexion is common in patients with previous fracture or osteoarthritis.

Supination
Normal = 90°, functional = 50°. This is rotation of the forearm with palm facing up.

Primary supinators

1. Biceps
   Musculocutanous nerve, C5,C6.
2. Supinator
   Radial nerve, C6.

Secondary supinator
Brachioradialis.

Pronation

Normal = 90°, functional = 50°. This is rotation of the forearm with the palm facing down.

Primary pronators

1. Pronator teres
   Median nerve, C6.
2. Pronator quadratus
   Anterior interosseous branch of median nerve, C8, T1.

Secondary pronator

Flexor carpi radialis.
Note: Loss of pronation and supination can result from fractures, arthritis, or dislocations.

Reflex testing

1. Biceps reflex, C5 nerve level
2. Brachioradialis reflex, C6 nerve level
3. Triceps reflex, evaluate the C7 nerve level.

MOTOR ASSESSMENT

First check active ROM. If a patient cannot perform the active test or there is a limitation in active ROM, then check passive ROM.

Normal active ROM

Flexion to 160°
Patient should be able to touch his/her shoulder normally.

Extension to 0–5°
Patient should be able to straighten elbow fully

Supination and pronation to 90°
Assess pronation and supination with elbow flexed at 90°.
Assess proximal and distal joint movement to help determine extent of injury.

1. Proximal: shoulder
2. Distal: wrist.

Compare flexion and extension of the right and left upper extremity. Compare pronation and supination of the right and left upper extremity – assess with arms at sides and elbow flexed to minimize shoulder movement.

COMMON SIGNS

OK sign

Inability to bring the tip of the thumb and the index finger together indicates injury to anterior interosseous nerve.

COMMON INJURIES

Tennis elbow

Epidemiology: very common; usually occurring in patients aged 35–50. Pathogenesis: injury probably due to repetitive strain of the common extensor origin at the lateral epicondyle.

Diagnosis: severe tenderness over lateral epicondyle at the attachment of forearm extensors. Ask patient to extend the elbow and perform extension of the wrist against resistance. Pain at lateral epicondyle is typical of tennis elbow. This test is usually done with elbow in extension.

Signs and symptoms: pain on the lateral elbow and difficulty holding heavy objects at arm's length.

Treatment: initially rest, heat, and physical therapy for stretching and gradual resumption of strengthening activities. A wrist splint can decrease stress of extensor tendons at the wrist. Steroid injection is reserved for patients with intractable pain.

Golfer's elbow

Not as common as tennis elbow and presents with pain in the medial epicondyle region at the site of attachment of forearm flexors. Test by asking the patient to flex the wrist against resistance. Pain in medial epicondyle is typical of golfer's elbow. The etiology is also repetitive stress activities but can be associated with a single traumatic incident. Golfer's elbow should not be confused with other causes of medial elbow pain, such as ulnar nerve compression.

Forearm fractures

A fall onto an outstretched hand can result in the fracture of ulna, radius or both. Although this can occur in any age group, it is more common in children. With any forearm fracture both the wrist and the elbow joint needs to be visualized on the radiograph. Fracture of the ulna may be associated with radial head dislocation (Monteggia fracture). Fracture of the radius may be associated with dislocation of the distal radioulnar joint in the wrist (Galazzi fracture).

Olecranon bursitis (a.k.a splunker's or student's elbow)

Epidemiology: common in carpet-layers and others who repeatedly traumatize the posterior aspect of the elbow joint; also common in RA.

Pathogenesis: swelling of the bursa.

Signs and symptoms: pain, but may be completely asymptomatic; nodular presence on posterior olecranon.

Treatment: empirical usually. Excision for cosmetic reasons only. If there is a possibility of septic elbow, drain and culture.

Nerve entrapment syndromes

All nerves of the upper extremity crossing the elbow can be compressed here.

- Median nerve: compression at the elbow is not as common as at the wrist (carpal tunnel syndrome). The nerve may be compressed by LLPF (**l**igament of Struthers; **l**acertus fibrosus –thickening of bicipital aponeurosis; **p**ronator teres; and **f**lexor digitorum superficialis)
- Ulnar nerve: arcade of Struthers
- Radial nerve.

Nursemaid's elbow (Fig. 4.2)

This is when the radial head is pulled out of the annular ligament as a result of traction injury.

Epidemiology: common in children under five years old; due to weak annular ligament not being fully formed.

Pathogenesis: due to traction of the arm; radial head slides out from under orbicular ligament.

Signs and symptoms: pain and limitation with supination; child presents with elbow tight at side not allowing the examiner to touch it.

Treatment: spontaneous reduction in 48 hours with rest or forced reduction via forced supination with pressure on the radius in the proximal direction. Apply pressure at brachial radialis with the thumb, supinate and flex, then feel pop under thumb when reduced.

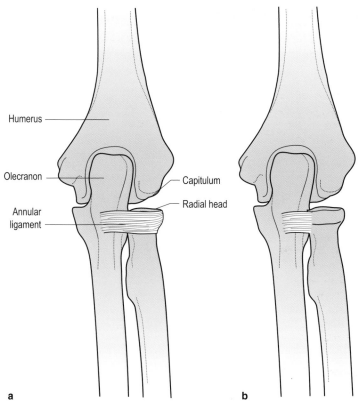

Humerus

Olecranon

Annular
ligament

Capitulum

Radial head

a

b

Fig. 4.2
Pulled elbow (nursemaid's elbow) (a) Normal (b) The radial head has been
pulled out of the annular ligament.

5

Wrist and hand

DESCRIPTION OF THE WRIST JOINT

The wrist joint is complex with radius, ulna and eight carpal bones (Fig. 5.1). The wrist has a dorsal and palmar surface as well as a radial (outer) and an ulnar (inner) border.

DESCRIPTION OF COMPONENTS

Wrist bones

Proximal row from radial to ulnar:

- Scaphoid
- Lunate
- Triquetrum
- Pisiform.

Distal row from radial to ulnar:

- Hamate
- Capitate
- Trapezoid
- Trapezium.

Hand bones (Fig. 5.2)

- Metacarpals
- Phalanges.

INSPECTION

Observe both hands at the same time for:

- Asymmetry
- Telescoping or shortening of the phalanges (i.e. psoriatic arthritis)
- Ecchymosis
- Edema

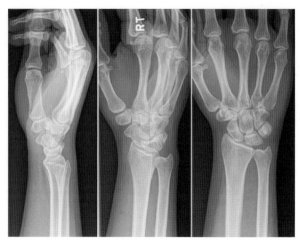

Fig. 5.1
Radiograph of the wrist

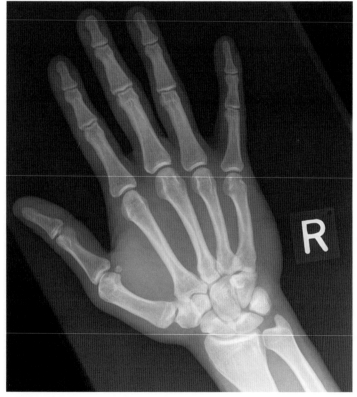

Fig. 5.2
Radiograph of the hand (anteroposteror view)

- Nodules
- Deformities: pitting, spooning, clubbing, swan neck deformity and boutonniere deformity (RA), mallet finger (Fig. 5.3)
- Color changes (i.e. cyanotic fingertips; pale or whitish finger nails in anemia; bruising, redness seen with cellulitis)
- Lacerations or scars.

PALPATION

Touching the patient's hands can help determine masses, joint effusions, areas of tenderness, crepitation, and clicking or snapping. Some specific areas that can be palpated include:

Radial styloid process: it is bordered by tendons of abductor pollicis longus and extensor pollicis brevis on the radial side and extensor pollicis longus on the ulnar side. Deep branch of the radial artery is occasionally palpable in the anatomical snuff box.

Anatomical snuff box: located slightly distal and dorsal to the styloid process of radius. Any tenderness on the floor of the anatomical snuff box suggests fracture of the scaphoid bone.

Scaphoid bone: represents the floor of anatomical snuff box and is the largest bone of the proximal row. It is the most commonly fractured carpal bone.

Bony enlargements

- Distal interphanlgeal joint (DIP): Herberden's nodes (osteoarthritis)
- Proximal interphalangeal joint (PIP): Bouchard's nodes (osteoarthritis).

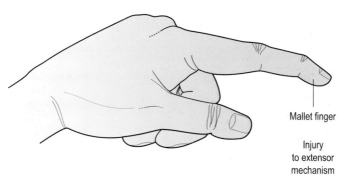

Mallet finger

Injury to extensor mechanism

Fig. 5.3
Mallet finger

Soft tissue palpation

Tendons of abductor pollicis longus and extensor pollicis brevis: a site for stenosing tenosynovitis (De Quervain's diseases), in which inflammation of these tendons causes pain when the tendons move.

Ganglion: on occasion a cystic, pea-sized swelling with a jelly-like consistency may develop on the dorsal or volar aspect of the wrist. It is not fixed to connective tissue and is not tender on palpation.

Palmaris longus: ask the patient to flex his wrist and touch the tips of his thumb and little finger together in opposition. The palmaris longus becomes prominent in the midline of the anterior aspect of the wrist.

Thenar eminence: situated at the base of thumb, the thenar eminence can be atrophied in compression of the median nerve since the median nerve innervates its muscles.

Hypothenar eminence (Fig. 5.4): situated at the base of the 5th finger, it can be atrophied in ulnar nerve palsy.

Palmar aponeurosis: extends to the base of fingers. Should be probed for palpable thickening in the form of nodules that are found usually on the ulnar side and may cause flexion deformity of the fingers (Dupuytren's contracture).

Fingers: palpate to find any tenderness or swelling in tufts of finger, which can be a sign of infection (felon). A handnail infection

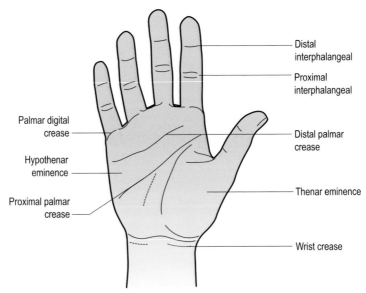

Fig. 5.4
Surface anatomy of the hand

or paronychia usually starts at the side of the nail and spreads around the nail base.

MOTOR ASSESSMENT

Both passive (examiner moving the joints) and active (patient moving) ROM (Fig. 5.5) should be documented. Pain with motion should be noted.

Normal active ROM

Wrist

Assess normal ROM by having the patient make a fist:

- Palmar flexion to 90°
- Dorsiflexion to 70°
- Normal ulnar deviation = 50°
- Normal radial deviation = 25°.

Fingers

MCP joints

- Palmar flexion to 90°
- Dorsiflexion to 30–45°.

PIP joints

- Palmar flexion to 100°
- Dorsiflexion to 0°.

DIP joints

- Palmar flexion to ± 90 °
- Dorsiflexion to 10°.

Finger abduction and adduction

Measured from axial line of the middle finger (see Fig. 5.5). Fingers are abducted almost 20° from the axial line.

Thumb motion

MCP joint:

- Extension to 20 °
- Abduction to 70°
- Adduction to 0°.

Interphalangeal joint

- Flexion to 50°
- Extension to 20°.

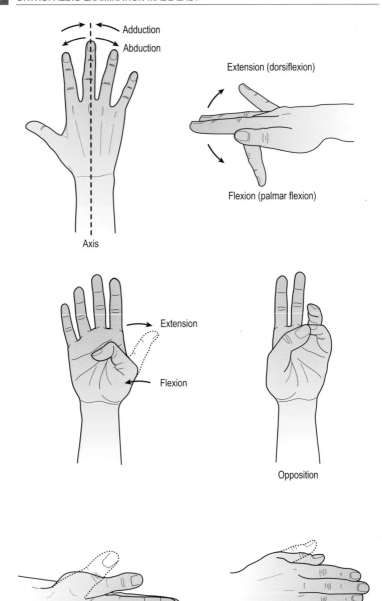

Fig. 5.5
Finger ROM

NEUROLOGICAL ASSESSMENT

Motor testing

Wrist extension: C6

- Extensor carpi radialis longus (radial nerve, C6, C7)
- Extensor carpi radialis brevis (radial nerve, C6, C7)
- Extensor carpi ulnaris (radial nerve, C6, C7).

Wrist flexion: C7

- Flexor carpi radialis (median nerve, C7)
- Flexor carpi ulnaris (median nerve, C7).

Fingers extension: C7

- Extensor digitorum communis (radial nerve, C7)
- Extensor indicis (radial nerve, C7)
- Extensor digiti minimi (radial nerve, C7).

Fingers flexion: C8

PIP joints

- Flexor digitorum profundis (ulnar nerve, C8, T1)
- Flexor digitorum superficialis (ulnar nerve, C7, C8, T1).

DIP joints

- Flexor digitorum profundis (ulnar nerve, C8, T1).

MCP joints
Lumbricals:

- Medial two lumbricals (ulnar nerve, C8, T1)
- Lateral two lumbricals (median nerve, C7).

Fingers abduction: T1

- Dorsal interossi (ulnar nerve, C8, T1)
- Abductor digiti minimi (ulnar nerve, C8, T1).

Fingers adduction: T1

- Palmar interossi (ulnar nerve, C8, T1).

Thumb extension

MCP joint

- Extensor pollicis brevis (radial nerve, C7).

Interphalangeal joint

- Extensor pollicis longus (radial nerve, C7).

Thumb flexion

MCP joint

- Flexor pollicis brevis (medial portion: ulnar nerve, C8, T1), (lateral portion: median nerve, C7).

Interphalangeal joint:

- Flexor pollicis longus (median nerve, C8, T1).

Thumb abduction

- Abductor pollicis longus (radial nerve, C7)
- Abductor pollicis brevis (median nerve, C6, C7).

Thumb adduction

- Adductor pollicis (ulnar nerve, C8).

Opposition of thumb and little finger

- Opponens pollicis (median nerve, C6, C7)
- Opponens digiti minimi (ulnar nerve, C8).

Sensation testing

The radial nerve innervates the dorsum of the hand on the radial side of the third metacarpal and dorsal surfaces of the thumb, index and middle fingers as far as the DIP joint. The web space between the thumb and index fingers are almost completely supplied by the radial nerve.

The median nerve innervates the radial portion of the palm and palmar surfaces of the thumb, index and middle fingers. It may innervate the dorsum of the terminal phalanges of these fingers. Its purest innervation area is on the palmar side of the tip of the index finger.

The ulnar nerve innervates the ulnar side of the hand, both palmar and dorsal surfaces. Its purest innervation area is on the palmar side of the tip of the little finger.

Sensation testing by neurologic level

See Figure 5.6.

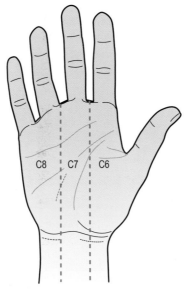

Fig. 5.6
Sensory supply to the hand

COMMON TESTS

Finkestein test

Instruct the patient to make a fist, with thumb tucked inside of other fingers. Then deviate the wrist to the ulnar side. If this movement causes pain on the radial side of the wrist, it is strong evidence of stenosing tenosynovitis (DeQuervain's tendonitis).

Phalen's test (Fig. 5.7a)

Palmar flex the patient's wrists to maximum degree, holding this position for at least one minute. If there is compression on the median nerve (carpal tunnel syndrome), the patient may feel tingling in the fingers.

Tinel's sign (Fig. 5.7b)

If you tap on the median nerve in the palmar side of wrist, the patient may feel a tingling sensation in the distribution of the median nerve in carpal tunnel syndrome.

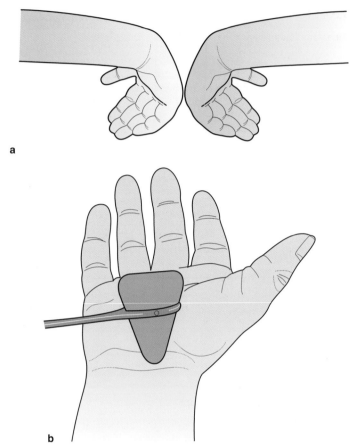

Fig. 5.7
Tests of the hand and wrist. **a.** Phalen's test; **b.**Tinel's sign

Allen test

This test is used to determine whether radial and ulnar arteries supply the hand with their full capacity or not. To perform this test, first press on the radial and ulnar arteries to obstruct blood flow and ask the patient to open and close his fist quickly several times to force venous blood flow out of the palm. Then, ask the patient to open his hand. The palm should be pale. Release one of the arteries at the wrist while you press the other. Normally the hand flushes immediately. If it flushes slowly, it is a sign of partially or completely occluded artery. Test the other artery to evaluate the blood flow in it.

COMMON INJURIES

Scaphoid (a.k.a carpal navicular) fracture

Epidemiology: common.
Pathogenesis: usually a fall onto outstretched hand.
Signs and sypmtoms: snuff box tenderness.
Treatment: need scaphoid view X-rays – full ulnar deviation.
Possible radial artery branch severance: recheck X-ray often to ensure healing, as there is an increased risk of avascular necrosis.

Carpal tunnel

Epidemiology: associated with edematous states and decreased nerve healing capabilities i.e. pregnancy, diabetes mellitus (DM), RA, hypothyroid and chronic heart failure (CHF).
Pathogenesis: impinged median nerve due to compression from inflamed tendons in the carpel tunnel.
Signs and symptoms: awake at night with parasthesias, e.g. a need to "shake out" the hands to relieve symptoms. Patients may have thenar atrophy, pain on pinch grip pain (test by having patient make an "okay" sign and the examiner pushes down on thumb). Sensation loss in median nerve distribution (thumb, first and half of second finger) may occur.
Diagnosis: reproduce symptoms with Tinel's or Phalen's sign.
Treatment: night brace or surgical decompression.

DeQuervian's tenosynovitis

Epidemiology: overuse of thumb with activities such as keyboarding.
Pathogenesis: tenosynovitis of abductor pollicis longus and extensor pollicis longus.
Signs and symptoms: pain over radial border of the wrist.
Diagnosis: Finkelstein's sign – the patient makes a fist with thumb inside fingers. This sign is positive if pain is felt on ulnar deviation. Occasionally crepitus may be felt in the tendons.
Treatment: Non-steriodal inflammatory medication, splint, and occasionally steroid injections.

Trigger finger

This occurs on the flexor tendon at A1 pulley; mostly only at fourth finger. The tendon flexes because flexor strength is greater than extensor strength, so it gets stuck.

If flexed without the strength to extend, this may develop into a Dupuytren's contracture. Pathology = palmar apeneurosis adhesions.

Gamekeeper's thumb

Epidemiology: injury to thumb.

Pathogenesis: sprain or rupture of ulnar collateral ligament of the thumb metacarpophalangeal (MCP) joint.

Signs and symptoms: pain in ulnar border of thumb; instability with full rupture.

Diagnosis: Gamekeeper's test – application of radial stress to the MCP joint of the thumb in full extension and 30° of the thumb.

Treatment: pain relief, splinting, and surgery for unstable joints with full rupture.

6

Hip and pelvis

DESCRIPTION OF THE JOINT

The hip joint is a large, deep ball and socket joint consisting of the femoral head articulating with the acetabulum (Fig. 6.1). The hip joint is extremely stable due to highly congruent bony contact and strong ligamentous support. The sacroiliac joint is immobile and therefore will not restrict movement, as would an injury to the hip joint. Pain in the pelvic girdle (Fig. 6.2) will likely be from one of five sources:

- Hip joint
- Soft tissues
- Pelvic bone
- Sacroiliac joint
- Referred pain from the lumbar spine.

Patients usually perceive their hip pain in the groin.

DESCRIPTION OF COMPONENTS

Bones
Pelvic girdle:

- Sacrum
- Pubic ramus
- Ilium.

Muscles

See Table 6.1.

Soft tissues

Iliofemoral ligament: a Y-shaped ligament, it is the strongest ligament in the pelvis. Arising from the anterior inferior iliac spine (AIIS) and the acetabular rim, it attaches to the intertrochanteric line. It prevents excessive extension.

Pubofemoral ligament: passes from the iliopubic eminence and obturator crest to the capsule on the inferior part of the neck of the femur. The ligament is tight in abduction and extension.

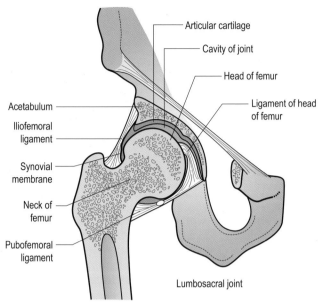

Fig. 6.1
Articulation of the femoral head and the acetabulum

Ischiofemoral ligament: arises from posteroinferior margin of acetabulum and passes to the capsule around the neck of the femur. It forms the zona orbicularis that keeps the loose capsule in good contact with the underlying retinacular fibers.

INSPECTION

It is very important to observe the patient as they walk into the office.

Gait

Observe the gait from side, front and behind. Assess stride length and stance on each leg. Signs of abductor deficiency (Trendelenberg gait), pain (antalgic gait), stiffness, and short leg become apparent during walking:

- Asymmetry:
  - Assess gluteal folds for signs of pelvic tilt
  - Observe the patient to see whether the AIISs are in the same horizontal plane or not
  - Observe the lumbar portion of the spine from the side. It normally exhibits a slight anterior curvature, or so-called lordosis. An absence of this slight lordosis suggests paravertebral muscle spasm. If there is a hyperlordosis the anterior abdominal muscles may be weak or there may be a fixed flexion deformity of the hip joint

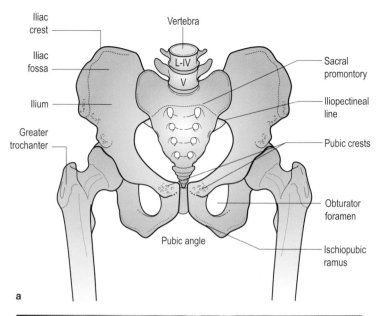

Iliac crest

Iliac fossa

Ilium

Greater trochanter

Vertebra

L-IV

V

Sacral promontory

Iliopectineal line

Pubic crests

Obturator foramen

Pubic angle

Ischiopubic ramus

a

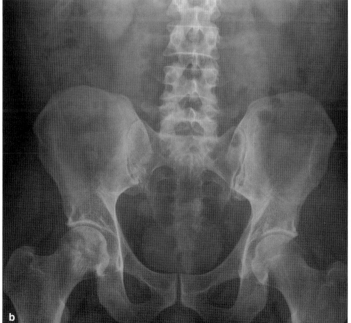

b

Fig. 6.2
Hip joint. a. Anatomy; b. Radiograph: anteroposterior view

Table 6.1
Muscles of the hip and pelvis

Muscles	Origin	Insertion
Psoas	Lumbar vertebra	Lesser trochanter
Iliacus	Iliac fossa	Lesser trochanter
Sartorius	ASIS	Medial tibial condyle
Quadriceps femoris (rectus femoris, vastus lateralis, vastus medialis, vastus intermedius)	Rectus from AIIS, and periacetabular region Vasti: upper femur	Tibial tubercle via patellar ligament
Adductor longus, adductor brevis	Pubic tubercle	Linea aspera
Adductor magnus	Ramus of pubis and ischium, ischial tuberosity	Linea aspera
Pectineus	Ramus of pubic bone	Upper part of linea aspera
Gluteus maximus	Ilium, sacrum, sacrotuberous ligament	Iliotibial tract
Gluteus medius	Ilium	Greater trochanter
Gluteus minimus	Ilium	Greater trochanter/ capsule
Piriformis	Sacrum	Greater trochanter
Obturator internus/gemelli/ quadratus femoris	Sacral tuberosity	Greater trochanter
Semitendinosus	Ischial tuberosity	Medial condyle of tibia
Semimembranosus	Ischial tuberosity	Medial condyle of tibia
Biceps	Ischial tuberosity (long head), linea aspera (short head)	Fibular head

- In infants check the skin folds in the hip region.
  The asymmetrical skin folds can be a sign of congenital
  dislocation of hip, muscular atrophy, pelvic obliquity or leg
  length discrepancy
- Color changes
- Lacerations
- Bruising
- Ecchymosis
- Edema
- Nodules
- Scars or sinuses.

PALPATION

Bony landmarks

- Anterior aspect: Anterior superior iliac spine (ASIS), iliac crest,
  greater trochanter, pubic tubercle
- Posterior aspect: posterior inferior iliac spine (PSIS), greater
  trochanter, ischial tuberosity, sacral prominence, sacroiliac joint.

Iliac crest
Palpate to check if there is any palpable enlargement. An enlargement in this area may be a neuroma in the cluneal nerve, which
sometimes occurs after taking an iliac bone graft.

ASIS
The ASIS is used as the most reliable bony landmark to assess limb
length. True limb length is measured from the ASIS to the malleolus.
Apparent limb length is measured from the umbilicus to the
malleolus.

Greater trochanter
Tenderness over the greater trochanter (GT) is indicative of bursitis
that may also present as hip pain.

SOFT TISSUE PALPATION

Femoral triangle
Defined by the inguinal crease superiorly, adductor longus muscle
medially and sartorius muscle ridge laterally, its floor is formed by
the thigh muscles. The femoral artery and lymph nodes are
superficial to iliopsoas muscle and psoas bursa and the hip joint lies
deep to it.

Inguinal ligament: located between ASIS and pubic tubercle.
Any unusual bulges along the course of this ligament may indicate
an inguinal hernia.

Femoral artery
Femoral nerve: passes lateral to femoral artery, not palpable
Femoral vein: passes medial to femoral artery, not palpable.

GT
Trochanteric bursa: lies in between the iliotibial band and the GT.

Sciatic nerve
Lies in the midpoint of the GT and the ischial tuberosity.

Hip and pelvic muscles
Flexor group: anterior quadrant

- Iliopsoas muscle: primary flexor of hip. Its abnormal contracture may lead to a flexion deformity of hip.
- Sartorius muscle: is the longest muscle of the body.
- Rectus femoris: is the only two-joint muscle in the anterior muscle group. It flexes the hip and extends the knee joint.

Adductor group: medial quadrant

- Gracilis muscle
- Pectineous muscle
- Adductor longus: the most superficial muscle and the only muscle of this group that is palpable
- Adductor brevis
- Adductor magnus.

Abductor group: Lateral quadrant

Gluteous medius: the main abductor of the hip.

Extensor group: posterior quadrant

Gluteous maximus: the primary hip extensor.
Hamstring muscles: consists of biceps femoris on the lateral side and semitendinosus and semimembranous on the medial side.

MOTOR ASSESSMENT

First measure active ROM (Fig. 6.3), then passive ROM. One hand can be rested on the contralateral ASIS to assess pelvic motion.

Measure hip flexion

The patient should be supine: have him grasp his bent knee and bring it towards his chest; stop when the contralateral hip rises or when the back is flat. Measure the angle. Normal hip flexion = 90–120°.

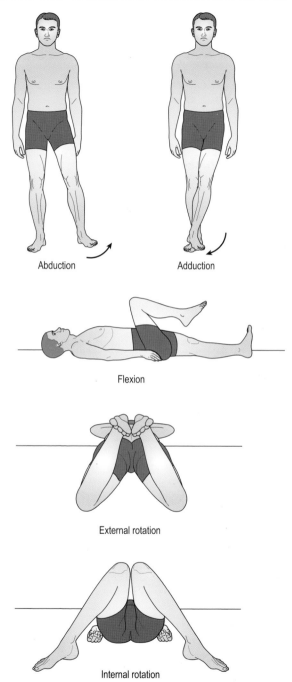

Abduction   Adduction

Flexion

External rotation

Internal rotation

Fig. 6.3
Hip ROM

Measure hip extension

The patient should be prone and should raise the entire leg; measure angle. Normal hip extension = 10–15° (30°).

Measure abduction/adduction

The patient should be supine: gently hold the ankle and abduct/adduct the leg. Stop when the ipsilateral pelvis begins to tilt. Hip abduction can also be measured accurately by measuring inter-malleolar separation during full abduction.

- Normal hip abduction = 45°
- Normal hip adduction = 30°.

Hip rotation

Decreases are seen with osteoarthritis. Internal femoral rotation: seated patient stabilizes knee and moves foot laterally. Normal = 35°.

An excessive femoral neck internal rotation may result from any increase in the normal anterior angulation of the neck of femur (anteversion), which is normally 15°. Infants usually have a greater degree of anteversion than adults.

External femoral rotation: seated patient stabilizes knee and moves foot medially. Normal = 45°. An excessive femoral neck external rotation may result from any decrease in the normal anterior angulation of the neck of femur (retroversion), which is normally 15°.

Rotation of the hip can also be measured with the patient lying prone.

Hints:

- Hip pain is described as 'groin pain' and often referred to the knee (especially in children)
- In obese (or very thin) young boys, slipped capital femoral epiphysis is a cause of hip pain. It results in retroversion of the femoral neck, so resulting in an excessive external rotation of hip – more than 50% bilateral within two years. Slip occurs at the growth plate and must be pinned to keep the plate intact
- Osteoarthritis can limit motion in all planes, but it most often limits internal rotation and abduction.

NEUROLOGICAL ASSESSMENT

Muscle testing

Adductor strength

Have the patient keep his feet together while you try to spread his legs apart.

- Primary adductor: adductor longus (obturator nerve, L2, 3, 4)
- Secondary adductors: adductor brevis, adductor magnus, and pectineus gracilis.

Abductor strength
Resist the patient's effort to spread legs apart.

- Primary abductor: gluteus medius (superior gluteal nerve, L5)
- Secondary abductor: gluteus minimus.

Flexor strength
The patient should be seated: resist the patient's effort to lift bent leg off the table against your resistance at the distal femur.

- Primary flexor: iliopsoas (femoral nerve, L1, 2, 3)
- Secondary flexor: rectus femoris.

Extensor strength
Ask the patient to lie prone and flex his knee to relax the hamstring muscles.

- Primary extensor: gluteus maximus (inferior gluteal nerve, S1)
- Secondary extensor: hamstrings.

Sensation testing

Test each neurological level that innervates dermatomes of the lower abdomen, pelvic region and thigh.

COMMON TESTS

Trendelenburg test (Fig. 6.4a)

With the patient standing, have them raise one knee. If the pelvis of the lifted side raises, this is a normal (negative) test. However, if the contralateral side of the pelvis raises, this is a positive Trendelenburg sign and indicates inadequate motor strength of the hip abductors.

Test for leg length discrepancy (Fig. 6.4b)

True leg length discrepancy
First, place the patient's legs in a precisely comparable position and measure the distance from ASIS to medial malleoli of the ankle. Unequal distance is a sign of true leg length discrepancy.

For determining a leg length discrepancy, ask patient to lie supine and flex his knee to 90°. If one knee appears higher than the other, the tibia of that extremity is longer.

Apparent leg length discrepancy

First perform the test for true leg length discrepancy (see above). On establishing that there is no true leg length discrepancy nor bony inequality, ask the patient to lie supine with his legs in a neutral position and measure the distance from umbilicus or xiphisternal junction to the medial malleoli of the ankle. Unequal distance signifies apparent leg length discrepancy, especially if there is not a true leg length discrepancy. Apparent leg length discrepancy may be caused by pelvic obliquity or adduction or flexion deformity in the hip joint.

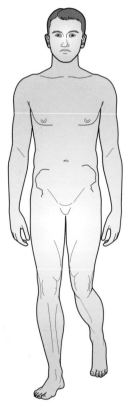 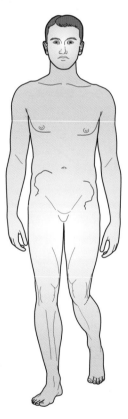

Negative
Standing on right leg.
Pelvis remains flat or elevated

Positive
Pelvis drops /tilts on the
affected extremity
(weak abductors; cannot
hold pelvis level)

a

Fig. 6.4
Tests for the hip. **a.** Trendelenberg test

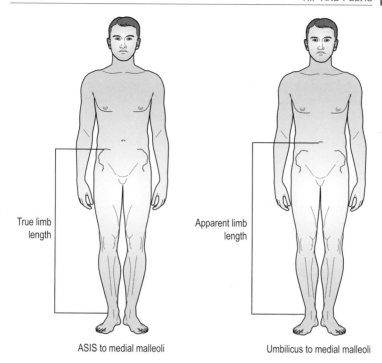

True limb length

ASIS to medial malleoli

Apparent limb length

Umbilicus to medial malleoli

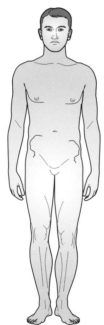

Pelvic obliquity may result in apparent (functional) limb length discrepancy

b

Fig. 6.4 *continued*
b. Leg length discrepancy

Thomas test for flexion contracture

Ask the patient to lie supine. Stabilize the pelvis by placing your hand under the patient's lumbar spine. Flex the hip and bring his thigh up onto his trunk. Normally, the lordosis of lumbar spine is flattened. Flex the other hip in a similar manner. Then ask the patient to hold his flexed hip on his chest and let the other hip extend until it is flat on the table. If the hip does not extend fully, the patient may have flexion contracture of the hip. Also, if the patient lifts his thoracic spine from the table or arches his back to reform the lumbar lordosis while lowering his other leg, it indicates a fixed flexion deformity.

Test for congenital dislocation of the hip

Ortolani's test

This test detects hips that are already dislocated. The hip is abducted while gently flexed and lifted with the fingers at GT. In a positive test, the reduction of the hip back into the acetabulum will be sensed and sometimes a clicking sound is audible.

Barlow's test

This test detects an unstable but located hip. The flexed thigh and knee are gently grasped in the hand with the thumb at lesser trochanter. The hip is adducted slightly and gently pushed posteriorly with the palm. In a positive test, the head of femur is subluxated over the posterior rim of the acetabulum.

Galeazzi's test

Flex the hips and knees of the child while lying in a supine position on a flat surface so the heels rest flat on the table. A dislocated hip results in a relative shortening of the thigh, shown by difference in knee height.

Telescoping

In a congenitally dislocated hip, pushing and pulling the hip in relation to the pelvis while the pelvis is stabilized with the other hand will result in a to-and-fro motion that is called telescoping.

Adduction contracture

In a dislocated hip the range of adduction is limited to 20° or less.

COMMON INJURIES

Hip dislocation

Epidemiology: history of high energy trauma e.g. motor vehicle accident or long fall.

Pathogenesis: dislocation of the femoral head from the acetabulum; most commonly posterior dislocation.

Signs and symptoms: pain, immobilization of the lower extremity and possible numbness.

Posterior dislocation: adducted, flexed and internally rotated.

Anterior dislocation: abducted, flexed and externally rotated.

Treatment – orthopaedic emergency:
– reduction after ruling out fractures
– crutch-assisted ambulation × 2 weeks
– weightbearing as tolerated.

Trochanteric bursitis

Epidemiology: history of lumbar spine disease, intra-articular hip pathology, and surgery or leg length inequalities.

Pathogenesis: inflammation of the trochanteric bursa.

Signs and symptoms: localized lateral hip pain; night pain; unable to lie on the affected side; distal radiation of pain or posterior radiation to buttock; pain my run down iliotibial band.

Treatment:
– NSAIDs
– iliotibial band stretching
– steroid injection.

Femoroacetabular impingement (Fig. 6.5)

This is a condition that can affect active young patients and results in early onset arthritis of the hip. There are two types: CAM impingement, more common in males, which occurs when the femoral head is out of round. During flexion the non-spherical femoral head causes an abuttment against the labrum and the underlying cartilage. This results in labral tear and cartilage flap separation. The other type is PINCER impingement, which is more common in females. The acetabulum is deeper than normal (protrusion, coax profunda) and hence the femoral neck abuts against the actebular rim. This also results in labral tear and cartilage flap separation.

Osteoarthritis of the hip

Epidemiology: > 70 years old.

Pathogenesis: degeneration of bony surfaces with increasing age.

Signs and symptoms: pain and decreased ROM.

Treatment: NSAIDs; arthroplasty if severe.

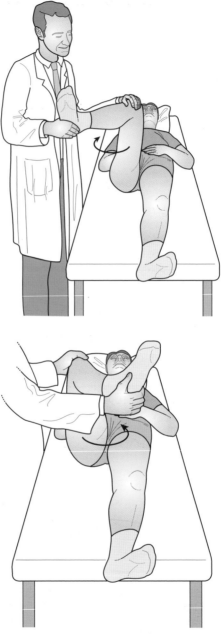

Fig 6.5
Femoroacetabular impingement test – Internal rotation of the hip is painful while external rotation does not cause much pain. The test is performed with patient lying supine, hip and knee both flexed to 90° and hip slightly adducted

7

Knee

DESCRIPTION OF THE JOINT

The knee joint is the largest joint in the body (Fig. 7.1). The knee is a synovial condylar joint with three bones (femur, tibia, and patella) creating movement at three articulating surfaces:

- Medial tibiofemoral
- Lateral tibiofemoral
- Patellofemoral.

The femoral condyles are rounded and lie perfectly on the tibial plateau. All of these articulating surfaces share a common synovial sheath, which extends around the lateral and medial sides of the patella, as well as proximally at its upper pole.

Although there are three articulations, there is no inherent stability at the knee joint. It therefore requires a complex ligamentous system to strengthen and secure the knee joint.

DESCRIPTION OF COMPONENTS

Bones

- Femur
- Tibia
- Patella – slides in a trochlear groove on the distal anterior femur equally between the medial and lateral epicondyle.

Muscles

The three medial hamstring muscles (sartorius, gracilis and semitendinosus) have a common insertion called the pes anserine or the 'goose foot'. Also of note is that each muscle has a different nerve supply, different origins and crosses two joints: the hip and the knee.

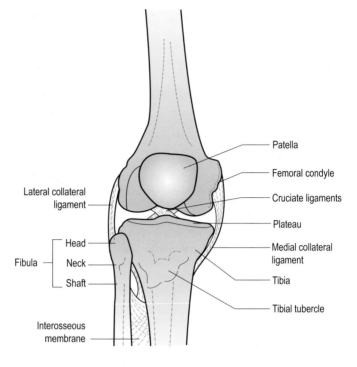

Patella

Femoral condyle

Lateral collateral ligament

Cruciate ligaments

Plateau

Head

Neck

Shaft

Fibula

Medial collateral ligament

Tibia

Tibial tubercle

Interosseous membrane

ai

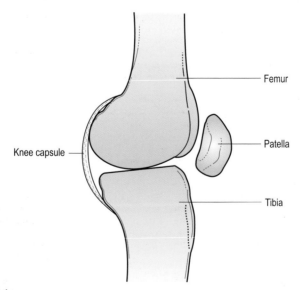

Femur

Knee capsule

Patella

Tibia

aii

Fig. 7.1
The knee joint. ai. Anteroposterior view; ii. Lateral view

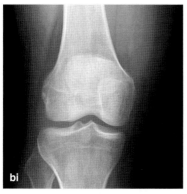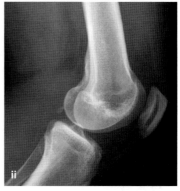

Fig. 7.1 *continued*
bi. Radiograph of anteroposterior view; **ii.** Radiograph of lateral view

Soft tissues

Lateral collateral ligament
The lateral collateral ligament extends from the lateral epicondyle to the head of the fibula distally.

Table 7.1
Knee muscles

Muscles	Origin	Insertion
Quadriceps femoris muscles, rectus femoris	Ilium, acetabulum	Patella
Quadriceps femoris muscles, vastus lateralis	Upper half of anterior intertrochanteric line, gluteal ridge, linea alba	Patella
Quadriceps femoris muscles, vastus medialis	Lower half of anterior intertrochanteric line, spiral line, internal supracondylar line	Patella
Quadriceps femoris muscles, vastus intermedialis	Anterior aspect of femoral shaft	Patella
Hamstring, semitendinosus	Ischial tuberosity	Upper subcut medial tibia
Hamstring, gracilis	Inferior pubic ramus	Upper subcut medial tibia
Hamstring, sartorius	ASIS	Upper subcut medial tibia

Medial collateral ligament

Broad and flat, the medial collateral ligament has a deep and superficial component, which extends from the medial femoral condyle to the medial surface of the tibia, straddling the semimembranous groove, distally.

Anterior cruciate ligament

The anterior cruciate ligament (ACL) runs obliquely from the anterior medial tibial plateau to the posterior lateral femoral condyle, preventing the tibia from sliding forward on the femur.

Posterior cruciate ligament

The posterior cruciate ligament (PCL) complements the ACL by running between the posterior lateral tibial plateau and lateral meniscus to the anterior medial femoral condyle, preventing the tibia from sliding backward on the femur.

The ACL and PCL lie within the intracondylar notch of the femur so that they are not trapped between the femur and tibia during knee flexion and extension.

Tendons

The quadriceps tendon secures the patella onto the anterior femur proximally. The patellar tendon secures the patella onto the tibial tuberosity distally.

Menisci

Lateral – posterior horn attaches to the femur; concave margin of anterior horn is unattached while convex portion is attached to the tibia via coronary ligaments.

Medial – no posterior horn attachment; anterior horn: concave margin is unattached while convex portion is attached to the tibia joint capsule.

Menisci also aid in maximal knee movement. These fibrocartilaginous discs cushion the femoral articulation with the tibia. They are C-shaped and composed of fibrous tissue. They are secured to the tibial plateau as well as loosely to the femur. During knee extension the menisci slide forward on the tibial plateau and are reshaped by compression allowing new relationships between the femur and tibia at each angle of extension. Meniscal tears have little chance of healing because they are vastly avascular, except for their peripheral edges.

The medial meniscus is more apt to injury as it is secured by the meniscofemoral ligaments (thickening of the capsule).

Bursae

- Suprapatellar pouch
- Pre-patellar bursa – between the patella and overlying skin

- Infra-patellar bursa
- Non-specific posterior bursa.

Bursae are numerous at the knee in the anterior and posterior portions of the knee joint. The suprapatellar bursa is a normal extension of the synovial compartment of the knee and can become prominent as a result of knee effusion.

The prepatellar bursa lies between the patella and the overlying skin. The bursa may become inflamed from kneeling (clergyman's knee).

The infrapatellar bursa is the region between the tibial tubercle, patellar ligament and the skin. This bursa may also become inflamed as a result of kneeling, but this is termed housemaid's knee.

Posteriorly large bursae exist that may become enlarged (Baker's cyst). These bursae communicate with the knee joint and can be distended with knee effusion.

INSPECTION

Observe patient as they walk into the examination room. Note any limp, stiff knee gait, use of walking aid, etc.

With the patient disrobed and standing assess for limb alignment: knock knee or genu valgum; bowed legs or genu varum; or hyper-extended knees or genu recurvatum (Fig. 7.2).

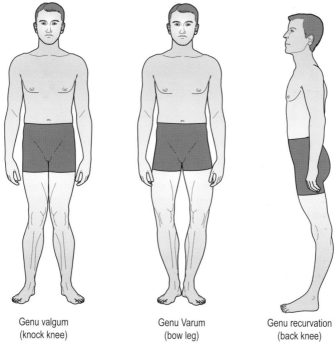

Genu valgum
(knock knee)

Genu Varum
(bow leg)

Genu recurvation
(back knee)

Fig. 7.2
Different gaits

Note any swelling:

- Prepatellar bursitis
- Infrapatellar bursitis
- Popliteal fossa cyst
- Pes anserinous bursitis
- Generalized swelling of the knee (hemorrhage, synovitis, infection).

Also look for:

- Muscle atrophy, especially of the extensor mechanism
- Color changes
- Lacerations
- Bruising
- Ecchymosis
- Scars and sinuses.

PALPATION

Start by feeling the temperature of the knee and always compare two sides. Warm knees may indicate acute injuries or infection. Locate the tibial tuberosity by traveling proximal on the flat surface of the medial tibia (shin) to the tibial tuberosity. From the tibial tuberosity follow further medially to the medial epicondyle. The lateral counterpart of the medial epicondyle is the lateral epicondyle. These three points form a triangle.

Feel the entire length of the patella. Palpate the joint line medially and laterally. The joint line is the first depression as you move your fingers up from the proximal tibia. Joint line tenderness indicates intra-articular pathology such as arthritis or meniscal tear.

Move the knee and feel for crepitus and patellar tracking. The patella should move in the trochlear groove. Note subluxation of patella. Crepitus signifies arthritis.

Locate the medial meniscus at the medial soft tissue depression at the proximal edge of the tibial plateau. Tenderness may signify tear. Locate the lateral meniscus with slight knee flexion at the proximal lateral edge of the tibial plateau. Again, tenderness may signify tear.

Palpate below the patella on both sides of the infrapatellar tendon for swelling; this is the infrapatellar bursa. Compare with the opposite knee for asymmetry.

Palpate the tibial tubercle to assess any swelling or pain that may be a sign of Osgood–Schlatter syndrome.

Palpate the pes anserine bursa on the upper medial aspect of the tibia, medial to the tibial tuberosity, to see whether there is any thickening, pain or effusion. Pes anserine bursa is the place of insertion of sartorius, gracilis and semitendinosus muscle tendons.

The popliteal artery is located deeply in the popliteal fossa behind the knee. To assess its pulse, ask the patient to relax his knee in flexion, so it may become accessible to palpation.

Assess ligamentous stability:

Collaterals: at full extension (0°) and with the knee flexed to 20° apply varus and valgus stress to the tibia while stabilizing the distal femur.

Cruciates: anterior drawer test (ACL), Lachman maneuver – described below, posterior drawer test (posterior cruciate ligament, PCL).

Menisci: McMurray's test, Apley compression-distraction test, squat test.

Measure the quadriceps girth at 15 cm proximal to the tibial tubercle in both extremities. Note any asymmetry.

MOTOR ASSESSMENT

First check the active then the passive ROM:

- Normal knee extension to 0°
- Normal knee flexion to 135°
- Normal knee internal and external rotation to 10°.

NEUROVASCULAR ASSESSMENT

Palpate pulses distally – dorsalis pedis and posterior tibial arteries. Test sensation and motor function of the foot.

Muscle testing

Extension
Primary extensors
Quadriceps femoris (femoral nerve, L2,3,4).

Flexion
Primary flexors
Hamstring muscles:

- Semimembranosus (tibial portion of sciatic nerve, L5)
- Semitendinosus (tibial portion of sciatic nerve, L5)
- Biceps femoris (tibial portion of sciatic nerve, S1).

Sensation testing

Test the dermatomes innervated by spinal nerve roots.

Reflex testing

Patellar reflex (knee jerk)
L2, 3, 4. Clinically, patellar reflex should be considered an L4 reflex, but it is innervated by more than one neurological spinal level.

Ankle reflex
S1.

COMMON TESTS

Apprehension test for patellar instability and subluxation (Fig. 7.3a)

Perform this with the patient sitting and supporting the lower leg to relax the quadriceps muscle. Place your thumb on the lateral femoral

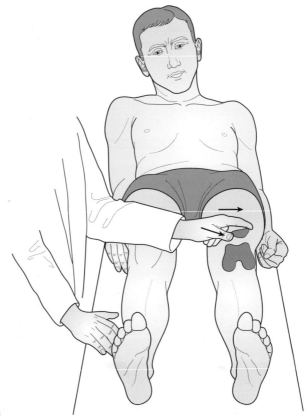

a

Fig. 7.3
Tests of the knee joint. **a.** Apprehension test

epicondyle while pushing the medial side of the patella laterally with your fingers – with instability the patella will subluxate. Next, watch as the patient flexes and extends the knee while sitting and look for an inverted 'J'- shaped motion of the patella as it moves proximally, indicating susceptibility to patellar subluxation.

Testing the medial collateral ligament

Secure the patient's ankle while he is lying supine. Place the other hand around the knee and push medially against the knee and laterally against the ankle in an attempt to open the knee in the inside. If there is a gap in the medial border of the knee joint, it shows that the medial ligament is damaged. This maneuver can be painful. Medial collateral ligament is critical in supporting the knee joint. Most injuries of ligaments occur in the medial side of knee.

Testing the lateral collateral ligament

Reverse the position of your hand and push the knee laterally in an attempt to open it on the outside.

Drawer test (Fig. 7.3b)

Place the patient in a supine position with the knee 90° flexed; sit on the patient's foot and grasp the proximal tibia with two hands – try to slide the tibia anteriorly to test the ACL stability and posteriorly to test the PCL stability; compare with the uninjured knee.

- Posterior drawer positive = PCL deficiency
- Anterior drawer positive = ACL deficiency.

Before trying the drawer test, palpate the hamstring tendons with the index fingers while both hands are around the proximal tibia.

Lachman test (Fig. 7.3c)

With the patient in a supine position with the knee flexed 20°, stabilize the distal thigh with one hand and grasp the proximal tibia with the other hand – have the 'V' of your distal hand just medial to the infra-patellar tendon – and try to pull the tibia forward. Positive Lachman is when the tibia can be pulled forward, which means ACL deficiency. Compare with the uninjured knee.

Pivot shift test

This test is designed to evaluate the integrity of ACL. While the knee is held in extension and the leg internally rotated, a valgus force is applied and the knee is flexed. Positive test is when the lateral tibial

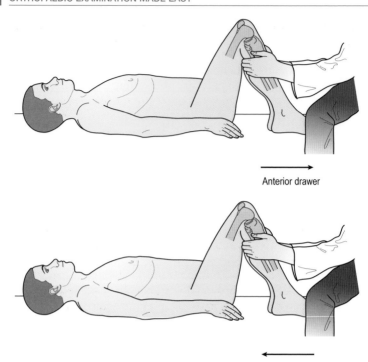

Anterior drawer

Posterior drawer

b

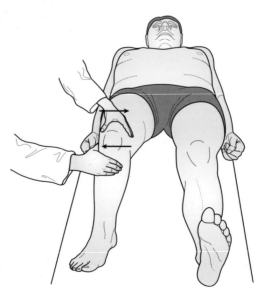

c   Lachman test

Fig. 7.3 *continued*
b. Drawer test; **c.** Lachman test

plateau shifts posteriorly and is reduced. During extension the tibia is anteriorly translated due to lack of restraint by the ACL.

McMurry test

Having the patient in a supine position with the hip and knee flexed; palpate lateral joint space with the fingers of one hand while alternating between internal and external rotation of the foot with the opposite hand. Severe pain associated with meniscal snap or crepitus will be felt with lesions of the posterior lateral or medial meniscal horns.

Squat test

Have the patient perform several repetitions of full squat with the feet and legs alternately fully internally and externally rotated as the squat is performed. Pain in medial or lateral side is suggestive of medial or lateral meniscal tear, respectively. Pain with lateral meniscal tear (lateral pain) is worse with the leg internally rotated and pain of medial menical tear is made worse with the leg externally rotated.

Apley compression tests (Fig. 7.3d)

Ask the patient to lie prone, with the leg flexed to 90°. While gently holding the thigh to stabilize, compress the heel and rotate the leg medially and laterally to evaluate the medial and lateral menisci. If this maneuver results in pain, it may be a sign of medial (pain in medial side of knee) or lateral (pain on lateral side of the knee) meniscal pathology.

Apley distraction test (Fig. 7.3e)

Ask the patient to lie prone, with the leg flexed to 90°, and while gently holding the thigh to stabilize, apply traction to the leg while rotating the tibia internally and externally. This maneuver reduces the pressure on menisci and puts strain on the medial and lateral collateral ligament. If this maneuver results in pain, it may be a sign of medial or lateral collateral ligament pathology.

Reduction click

This maneuver is applicable for those patients who have a locked knee due to torn or dislocated menisci. With the patient in the supine position, flex the knee and internally and externally rotate the knee to reduce the displaced or torn menisci. It will unlock the knee and permit full extension.

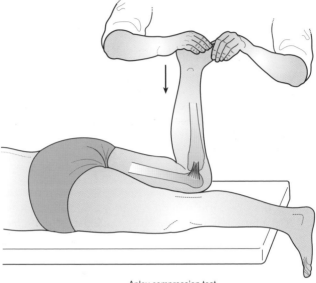

Apley compression test

d

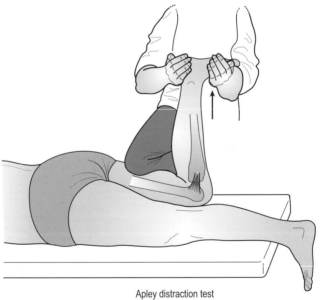

Apley distraction test

e

Fig. 7.3 *continued*
d. Apley compression test; **e.** Apley distraction test

Ober test (Fig. 7.3f)

The patient lies on the uninvolved side with the lower knee flexed to help reduce lumbar lordosis. The examiner lifts the upper flexed or extended leg at the ankle while stabilizing the pelvis with the other hand, then abducts and extends the hip allowing the iliotibial band (ITB) to move posteriorly over the GT. The examiner then slowly lowers the upper leg. If the leg drops to the table, the test is negative; if it remains abducted, the test is positive. It is extremely important in performing this test to hold the patient's pelvis and keep it at a right angle to the table while moving the involved side.

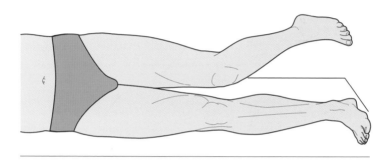

Positive

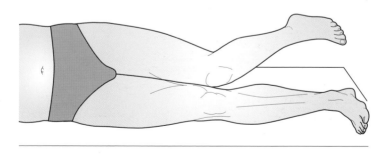

Negative

f

Fig. 7.3 *continued*
f: The Ober test

Knee joint effusion test (Fig. 7.3g)

Gently extend the knee and ask the patient to relax the quadriceps muscle, then push the patella into the trochlear groove and quickly release it. In large amounts of joint effusion, you can see the forced flow of fluid to the sides of joint, then the flowing back of the fluid which forces the patella to rebound (ballotable patella).

In minor effusions, extend the knee and milk the fluid from the suprapatellar pouch and lateral side into the medial side and tap gently over the fluid, which will create fullness on the lateral side.

Active quadriceps test

Place the patient supine and have the knee extended with the extensor mechanism relaxed. Hold the patella and gently press it into the trochlear groove. Ask the patient to contract the quadriceps. Patients who have cartilage lesion behind the patella, as in osteoarthritis or osteochondritis dissecans, usually feel pain in the patella region.

COMMON CONDITIONS
ACL tear

Epidemiology: history of twisting injury; usually associated with athletes; females are affected more than males.

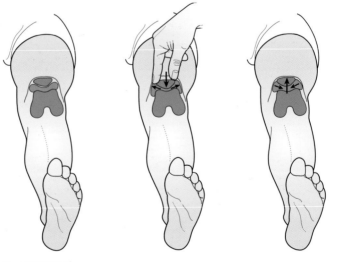

g

Fig. 7.3   *continued*
g. The knee joint effusion test

Pathogenesis: traumatic rupture of the primary knee anterior and rotational stabilizer.

Signs and symptoms: popping sensation at time of injury, effusion, painful ROM and profound difficulty ambulating.

Treatment, depending on patient age and activity level:

- Rest, Ice, Compression, Elevation (RICE) and NSAIDs
- Knee immobilizer
- Possible surgical reconstruction.

Meniscal tear

Epidemiology: history of twisting knee injury or older patients with degenerative tear and no history of injury.

Pathogenesis: traumatic or degenerative tear of the medial or lateral menisci.

Unhappy triad: medial meniscal tear may be associated with ACL and MCL tear due to the mechanism of injury – lateral clipping injury.

Signs and symptoms: able to ambulate followed by acute onset of swelling and stiffness; late surgery may include popping, clicking or locking.

Treatment:

- RICE and NSAIDs
- Possible surgical debridement if popping, clicking or locking continues.

Collateral ligament sprains

Epidemiology: history of valgus force without rotation (MCL), pure varus producing force on the knee (LCL).

Pathogenesis: traumatic rupture of the primary knee medial or lateral stabilizer.

Signs and symptoms: able to ambulate after injury; localized swelling and stiffness and localized (medial or lateral) pain and tenderness.

Treatment:

- Grade I: stretch, RICE and NSAIDs
- Grade II: partial tear – hinged brace; weightbearing as tolerated
- Grade III: complete tear – hinged brace; gradual return to weightbearing in four weeks.

8

Foot and ankle

DESCRIPTION OF THE JOINT

The ankle is a hinged joint with movement in the plantar flexion and dorsiflexion planes (Fig. 8.1). It is described as a mortice and because of its natural congruency has an excellent inherent bony stability. The subtalar joint (between calcaneus and talus) allows inversion and eversion. Numerous tendons and ligaments surround the ankle (Fig. 8.2). The position of each tendon and ligament gives a good clue regarding their function. For example, peroneal tendons located behind the lateral maleolus are important for eversion of the foot. The large and strong Achilles' tendon is the most important plantar flexor of the ankle. The foot is divided into three parts: hindfoot (talocalcaneal, talonavicular and calcanocuboid joints), midfoot (joints between all the other tarsal bones and the tarsometatarsal joints), and forefoot (all metatarsophalangeal joints) (Fig. 8.3).

Ligaments

There are a group of ligamentous structures that provide stability for the ankle joint:

Lateral ligament complex: has three parts which all arise from the fibula. The central portion of the ligament is attached to the calcaneus (calcaneofibular – CFL) while the anterior talofibular (ATFL) and posterior talofibular (PTFL) portion attach to the talus. These ligaments, particularly ATFL, are commonly injured during inversion ankle sprains.

Medial ligament complex: is triangular in shape and hence is called the deltoid ligament. It has deep layers that connect the medial malleolus (distal tibia) to talus and the superficial part that connects the tibia to the calcaneus and navicular bone. The spring ligament is composed of strong fibers of the medial complex that attach calcaneus to the navicular bone.

Tibiofibular ligaments: the inferior tibiofibular ligaments (anterior and posterior) fibers attach tibia to fibula. These are assisted by the interosseous membrane.

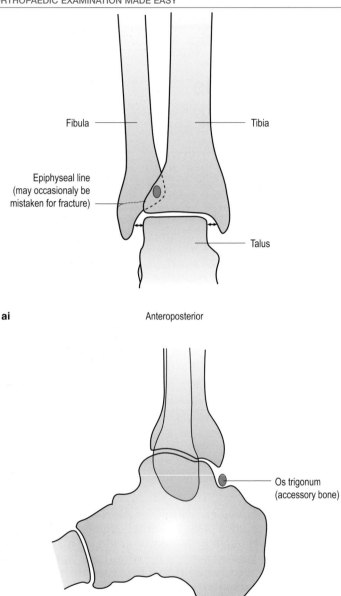

Fig. 8.1
The ankle joint. **ai.** Anteroposterior view: note symmetry in mortice (arrows). Distance of talus from tibia and fibula should be the same on true AP X-ray. Also, note overlap of tibia and fibula ('●'). This region, called syndesmosis, contributes to stability of the ankle. Separation of syndesmosis will result in reduced area of overlap; **ii.** Lateral view: os trigonum should not be mistaken for fracture

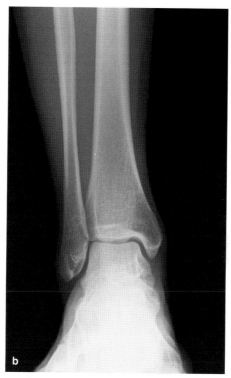

Fig. 8.1
b. Radiograph (anteroposterior view)

INSPECTION

Shoes

In many cases, the shoe is a literal showcase for certain disorders. The shoes of a person with flat feet will have broken medial counters; the shoes of a patient with toe-in show excessive wear on the lateral side; and the shoes of a patient with a drop foot display scuffed toes from scraping the floor in swing phase of walking. Hallux valgus (bunion) deformity usually causes a notable prominence in the front of the shoe on the medial side (Fig. 8.4).

Asymmetry

Assess the posture of the foot with patient sitting.

Edema

Look at the contour of the foot. Edema causes loss of all anatomical contours and creates stretched skin (loss of normal creases). There are

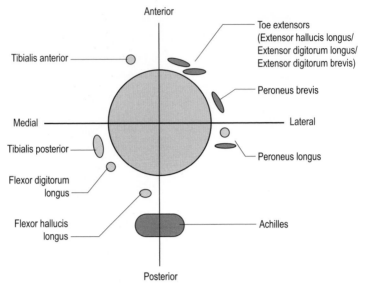

Fig. 8.2
The arrangement of the tendons around the ankle

numerous causes for ankle edema: mostly, and especially if bilateral, it is likely to be systemic causes, such as heart failure.

Deformities

There are many conditions that can result in deformity of the foot and ankle. Look for hallux valgus (bunion), hammer toe (Fig. 8.5a), claw toe (Fig. 8.5b), overlapping toes, high arched foot (pes cavus) (Fig. 8.5c), flat foot (pes planus), callosity or skin thickening in the areas of abnormal weightbearing.

Skin

Look at the skin carefully to note any previous scars, color changes (vascular problems or skin lesions), lacerations, bruising, and ecchymosis. Feel for any temperature difference. Ensure you look at the soles of the feet, web spaces (between the toes), and carefully examine the nails. Some serious pathologies such as melanoma may present in these spaces and can on occasions resemble subungal hematoma (bleeding under the nail). Another example of a serious condition is Kaposi's sarcoma (a condition seen in patients with AIDS), which can present on the sole of the foot. Athlete's foot (tinea pedis) presents in the web spaces.

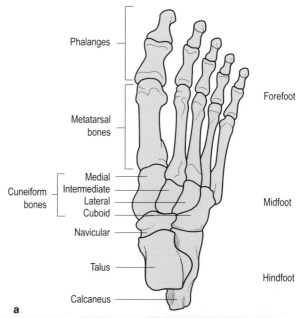

Phalanges

Metatarsal
bones

Forefoot

Cuneiform
bones

Medial
Intermediate
Lateral
Cuboid

Navicular

Talus

Calcaneus

Midfoot

Hindfoot

a

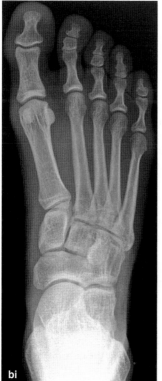

bi

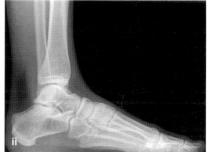

ii

Fig. 8.3
The foot

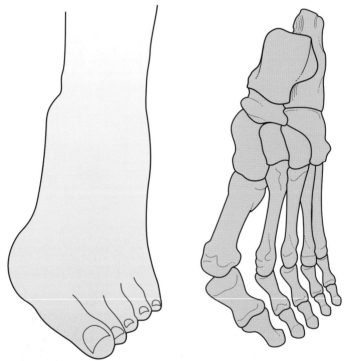

Fig. 8.4
Hallux valgus

PALPATION

Begin your palpation in a systematic manner. Start from the ankle and move distally. First assess the anterior joint line for swelling or tenderness. The joint line can be felt as a depression where the tibia ends. Dorsiflexion of the foot opens up the joint space and allows palpation of the anterior part of the talus. Other bones and their neighboring joint can all be felt in a systematic manner. Again feel all these for tenderness, deformities, bone spurs, and swelling. Ensure you feel the entire length of each metatarsal and the phalanges. Do not forget to palpate the tendons for tenderness, swelling and possibly discontinuity (ruptures). Start with the Achilles' tendon, feel anterior tendons (especially extensor hallucis longus, EHL), medial tendons (especially posterior tibialis), and the peroneals behind the lateral malleolus.

Some important landmarks

Head of the first metatarsal bone

The head of the first metatarsal bone is the site of the common condition, hallux valgus. In hallux valgus the first metatarsal shaft is medially

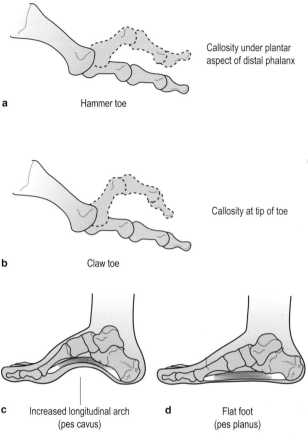

Callosity under plantar aspect of distal phalanx

a Hammer toe

Callosity at tip of toe

b Claw toe

c Increased longitudinal arch (pes cavus)

d Flat foot (pes planus)

Fig. 8.5
Abnormalities of the foot and ankle. **a.** Hammer toe; **b.** Claw toe; **c.** Pes cavus; **d.** Pes planus

angulated and the surrounding soft tissue at the head of this bone is swollen. This area appears reddened and is commonly called a bunion. Gout usually presents as pain and tenderness in the first metatarsophalangeal joint (so-called podagra).

Head of the fifth metatarsal bone
A bursa (fluid-filled space) exists in this area that can sometimes become inflamed. The overlying skin can also become red and tender. This condition is called tailor's bunion (as tailors used this aspect of the foot to run the pedal of their sewing machine) or bunionette (little bunion).

Base of fifth metatarsal

The tendon of peroneous brevis inserts into this region. On occasions avulsion fracture of this bone may occur during inversion injury.

Navicular bone

Tenderness over the prominence (tubercle) of the navicular bone is seen in patients with avascular necrosis of this bone (Kohler's disease).

Deltoid ligament

Medial collateral ligament of the ankle is palpable just inferior to the medial malleolus. This ligament can be sprained or torn during eversion injury of the ankle.

Posterior tibial tendon

This tendon just behind the medial malleolus can become swollen and tender that if long-standing can result in flat foot deformity.

Posterior tibial artery

The posterior tibial artery passes posterior to the medial malleolus with the tendons of tibialis posterior (known as 'Tom'), flexor digitorum longus ('Dick'), flexor hallucis longus ('Harry') and the posterior tibial nerve. Its pulsation can be palpated in a relaxed, non-weightbearing position by pressing the fingers gently into the posterior region of the medial malleolus.

Long saphenous vein

Immediately visible anterior to medial malleolus, the long saphenous vein is a site for i.v. infusion and venous cut down.

Dorsalis pedis artery

Lying between the first and second metatarsal bones on the dorsum of the foot the dorsalis pedis artery's pulses are easily detected. Reduced pulse is seen in vascular diseases but this artery is absent in 15% of the normal population.

Achilles' tendon

The Achilles' tendon is palpable from the lower third of the calf to the calcaneus bone. In cases of ruptured tendon, a gap is detected and pain is elicited during palpation of the tendon. There are two bursae in this region. One is located anterior to the Achilles' tendon – the retrocalcaneal bursa. The other lies between the Achilles' tendon and the overlying skin and is called calcaneal bursa. Pain is elicited if there is a bursitis in this area.

Fibular head

On occasions injury to the ankle results in fracture of the fibular head (Maisonneuve injury). The impact of the injury disrupts the interossous membrane between the tibia and the fibula with the exiting force at the fibular head resulting in fracture.

ROM

First, measure active ROM, then evaluate the passive ROM. Compare the ROM to the contralateral side. Reduced motion may be the result of degenerative joint disease (arthritis), fractures, swelling, or voluntary guarding because of pain. Feel for crepitations (arthritis) during motion of the joint. The position of the knee may affect ankle ROM. For example, flexion of the knee may improve dorsiflexion in patients with tight Achilles' tendon.

Expected ROM

- Ankle dorsiflexion to 20°
- Ankle plantar flexion to 50°
- Subtalar inversion and eversion of 5° each
- Forefoot adduction to 20°
- Forefoot abduction to 10°
- First metatarsophalangeal joint:
  – flexion to 45°
  – extension to 70–90°.

NEUROVASCULAR ASSESSMENT
Motor

Ask the patient to move the foot and the ankle in each direction against resistance. The following outlines the muscle groups that are responsible for each motion with the foot in neutral. Some of these tendons can be isolated if the foot is placed in the starting position of eversion or inversion. For example, posterior tibialis becomes the main muscle responsible for plantar flexion when the foot is placed in inversion.
  Dorsiflexion:

- Tibialis anterior (deep peroneal nerve, L4,5)
- Extensor hallucis longus (deep peroneal nerve, L5)
- Extensor digitorum longus (deep peroneal nerve, L5).

Plantar flexion:

- Peroneal longus and brevis (superficial peroneal nerve, S1)
- Gastrocnemius and soleus (tibialis nerve, S1,2)
- Flexor hallucis longus (tibial nerve, L5)
- Flexor digitorum longus (tibial nerve, L5)
- Tibialis posterior (tibial nerve, L5).

Eversion is mostly done by peroneals and inversion performed by the posterior tibialis.

Sensation

Evaluation of the sensation necessitates removal of shoes, stockings, pantyhose (tights) or trousers so that the examination is directly against the skin and can be extended to the knees. Sensation may be quickly assessed by touch. On occasions, and especially if sensory deficit is detected, detailed sensory examination might be necessary. In patients with diabetic neuropathy, for example, special filaments (Semmes–Weinstein) may be used to assess sensation. Proprioception, vibration, and detailed examination of the other sensory modalities are necessary for the select group of patients with neurological disorder. High arch foot (pes cavus) can present as part of a neurological disorder (such as Friedreich's ataxia) and should alert the examiner to the need for a thorough evaluation. The level of dermatomal distribution around the foot and ankle is shown (Fig. 8.6).

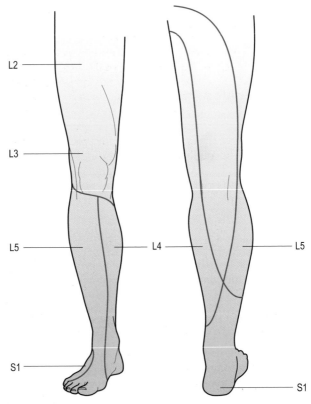

Fig. 8.6
Dermatomal distribution around the foot and ankle

Reflex testing

Achilles' tendon reflex – S1.

Vascular status

Feel for dorsalis pedis and posterior tibialis pulse. Peripheral vascular disease should particularly be suspected in heavy smokers, diabetics, and hypertensive patients. Venous insufficiency may present with dusky blue skin and ulcerations, mostly around medial malleolus. Capillary refill should also be assessed. Patient with non-palpable pulses need Doppler ultrasound and ankle brachial index (ABI) measurement.

GAIT

Once you are done with the examination of the patient sitting, ask the patient to stand. First inspect the overall alignment of the lower extremity and look for signs of genu varus or genu valgum. Assess to see if both feet are touching the ground (plantigrade). Limb length discrepancy or short Achilles' tendon may result in one heel not reaching the ground. With the patient standing inspect the ankle and the feet from the sides, behind and the front. Inspect the posterior heel for evidence of valgus (eversion) or varus (inversion) deformity. Look for evidence of high or flat arch in each foot. Ask the patient to stand on their heel (they will be unable to do so if there is a problem with the Achilles' tendon) or to stand on their tiptoes (unable if there are posterior tendon problems). Then ask the patient to walk with and without shoes and carefully inspect.

SOME COMMON TESTS

Anterior draw test

Similar to the anterior drawer test in the knee, it is used to diagnose anterior instability of the ankle that may arise because of ATFL insufficiency. To perform this test, the lower tibial is stabilized with one hand (left hand for a right-handed examiner) while the other hand holds and pulls the calcaneus forward (anterior). Anterior motion that is greater than the uninjured side (and usually more than three mm) is considered positive and may signify ATFL incompetence.

Valgus (eversion) stress

This tests the integrity of the medial ligamentous complex (deltoid ligament). The test is performed by stabilizing the lower tibia in one hand, while holding and everting the calcaneus with the other hand.

A palpable gap medially and excessive eversion may be the result of deltoid ligament injury (incompetency).

Forefoot adduction correction test

This is used to determine if any treatment for club foot is needed. If an adducted forefoot of an infant can be abducted beyond the neutral position, no treatment will be necessary, but if the adduction is not correctable or is just partially correctable, cast correction is necessary.

Homan's sign

Used as a diagnostic test for possible deep venous thrombosis (DVT), the test for Homan's sign is performed by forcibly dorsiflexing the patient's ankle. Pain in the calf is sign of a positive test and possible pointer for DVT. Many have questioned the value of this test.

Thompson's test (Fig. 8.7)

Thompson's test is used to evaluate the Achilles' tendon and the gastrocnemius and solus muscles. Ask the patient to kneel on the edge of the bed and have their feet hang free. Then squeeze the calf muscles and look at the feet. Absence of plantar flexion of the foot with calf muscle compression is a sign of Achilles' tendon rupture.

Foot drop

Lack of ability to dorsiflex the foot and/or the toes is a sign of injury to the anterior compartment muscles or the nerve innervating these muscles. Foot drop is relatively common and should alert the examiner to the presence of lumbar spine disorder, sciatic nerve injury (that can occur with surgery), or conditions affecting the anterior compartment muscles, such as compartment syndrome. Patients who are unable to walk on their heels have weakness of dorsiflexion.

COMMON CONDITIONS
Ankle sprains

Epidemiology: soft tissue injuries to the ankle are extremely common and can affect any age group.

Pathogenesis: most of these are inversion injuries resulting in sprain (incomplete tear) of lateral ligaments. On occasion, medial ligament injury can also occur. When there is complete rupture of the ligaments that fail to heal, instability of the ankle may result.

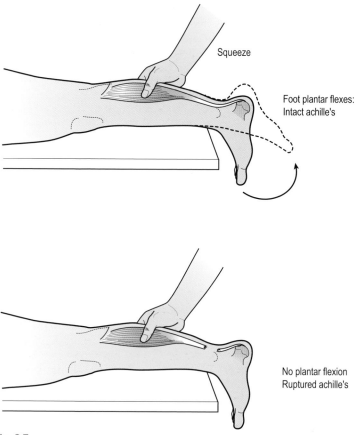

Fig. 8.7
Thompson's test

Signs and symptoms: pain, and inability to weight bear in some cases, are the main complaint. The ankle swells up and the swelling may be associated with areas of ecchymosis and bruising. Palpation of the ligaments especially ATFL is tender.

Ottowa ankle rule: this is used by some institutions to determine on which patients ankle radiographs should be ordered. The criteria are:

- No weightbearing x 4 steps at time of injury or at the time of examination
- Bony tenderness around medial or lateral malleolus
- Positive squeeze test: fibula and tibia pushed together by examiner at about the shin, creating pain at the ankle

- Stress test for lateral ligament tear of the ankle: grasp the heel and forcibly but gently invert the foot, feeling for any opening-up of the lateral side of the ankle between tibia and talus (Fig. 8.8).

Treatment: most are pure ligamentous injuries and may be treated with PRICE (Pain control, Rest, Ice, Compression, and Elevation). Fractures may require surgical fixation.

Achilles' tendon rupture

Epidemiology: this condition can affect any age group but is more common in middle age and can occur in healthy adults with no previous Achilles' tendon problems. Degenerative changes in the tendon with age, and long-standing inflammation of the tendon, especially if treated with steroid injections, are some of the predisposing factors.

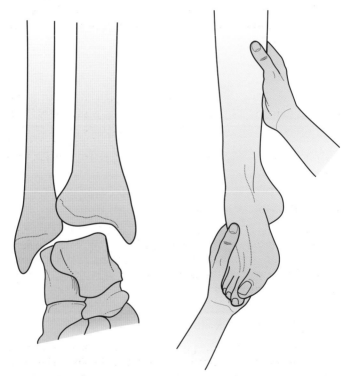

Fig. 8.8
Stress test for lateral ligament rupture – heel is grasped and forcibly inverted. Opening up of the lateral side of the ankle between tibia and fibula signifies rupture of the lateral ligamentous complex. If in doubt, a radiograph is taken to confirm

Pathogenesis: sudden and forceful plantar flexion and contraction of the tendon results in rupture. This should be distinguished from plantaris rupture that also occurs by the same mechanism. Plantaris rupture does not result in noticeable weakness of plantar flexion.

Signs and symptoms: the patient usually feels the rupture and might even hear the sound. Most patients describe the tear as a feeling of being kicked hard in the heel. Swelling around the rupture, tenderness, and loss of tendon integrity may be palpable. Thompson's test may be positive and there may be loss of power in plantar flexion.

Treatment: most are treated by surgical repair, although conservative treatment may also be viable.

Hallux valgus

Hallux valgus is a common condition affecting the great toe. The first metatarsal shifts into varus, sesamoid bones under the first meta-tarsophalangeal (MTP) joint subluxate laterally and the proximal phalanx is pulled into valgus. The process results in prominence of the first MTP joint.

Tenosynovitis

Tenosynovitis is an inflammatory condition often affecting the tibialis posteror or the peroneous longus tendon. Patients present with pain and swelling. A puffy swelling along the length of the tendon may be palpable. If long-standing, tenosynovitis could result in tendon rupture and incompetence. Flat foot may result from posterior tibialis tendon dysfunction (PTTD).

Osteochondritis dessicans

This condition commonly affects adolescents and the young. It presents with pain and, occasionally, swelling of the ankle. The feeling of something 'catching' in the ankle may also be present if free fragments float around the joint. This is usually treated by surgery to excise or re-attach the free fragments.

Snapping peroneal tendon

This condition presents with pain and the patient is usually able to feel the tendons ride over the lateral malleolus. The tear in the peroneal retinaculum allows the tendon to subluxate anteriorly. Treatment is usually by surgery and repair of the retinaculum.

Heel spur

This is an inflammation of the bursa overlying the calcaneus bone in the plantar surface. Palpation of this area with a gentle pressure causes pain.

Hammer toes

Hammer toes are defined as hyperextension of the metatarsophalangeal and distal interphalangeal joints and flexion of the proximal interphalangeal joint (see Fig. 8.5a).

Claw toes

Claw toes are defined as hyperextension of the metatarsophalangeal joints and flexion of the proximal and distal interphalangeal joints (see Fig. 8.5b).

Ingrown toenail

Ingrowing toenails involve the medial and lateral aspect of the toenails, causing infection and swelling in the adjacent soft tissue.

Corns

Corns are found most often between the fourth and fifth toes and are soft because of moisture between the toes. They may be tender on palpation.

Flat foot

The foot has longitudinal and transverse arches. The arches are created and supported because of the special shape and arrangement of the bones, constraint of the ligaments, and the dynamic pull of the muscles. Flat foot deformity results from disruption of any of these factors. Posterior tibial tendon dysfunction, either because of trauma or inflammation, is the most common and important cause of flatfoot deformity. Ligament rupture, fracture and deformities of bone can all conceivably result in flat foot deformity. There is a genetic component as foot arches may fail to develop in some people.

Arched foot (pes cavus) Figure 8.5c

Abnormally high longitudinal arches are produced as a result of imbalance in the dynamics that control and maintain the arches. Pes cavus is an abnormal finding and should always be investigated. Friedreich's ataxia, polio, spastic diplegia and spina bifida are examples of some conditions that may result in pes cavus.

Kohler's disease

This is osteochondritis of the navicular bone occurring in children between the ages of 5–7 years. The navicular bone shows increased density on the radiographs.

Morton's neuroma

This is a painful mass-like lesion occurring mostly between the third and fourth metatarsal heads but it can also occur between the second and third metatarsal heads. Morton's neuroma is not actually a true neuroma but a perineural fibrosis and nerve degeneration around the plantar digital nerve. The condition presents as pain in the affected web space. Clinical examination may reveal tenderness in the region of the neuroma. MRI may be used to diagnose the condition.

Plantar fasciitis

Epidemiology: 40–60 years old; status post heel trauma.
Pathogenesis: Excessive activities especially while carrying weight (e.g. waiters). Association with inflammatory arthropathy, such as Rieter's disease.
Signs and symptoms: tenderness at anteromedial calcaneus, the origin of plantar fascia; burning or aching sensation, most severe in morning.
Treatment: heel pad; NSAIDs; stretching.

Anterior talofibular ligament tear/sprain at inversion injury is the most common ankle injury with base of fifth metatarsal involvement.
Plantar fascitis is heel pain due to inflammation; treat with stretching heel cords.

Rocker bottom foot

Otherwise known as congenital vertical talus, rocker bottom foot is irreducible dislocation of the navicular on the talus. Clinically the talar head becomes prominent on the medial side, the sole is overtly convex, the forefoot is abducted and dorsiflexed, and the hindfoot is in equinovarus (Persian slipper foot). Patients may demonstrate a 'peg-leg' gait (awkward gait with limited forefoot pushoff). This condition is a common cause of rigid flatfoot. Vertical talus is occasionally associated with chromosomal abnormalities, myeloarthropathies, or neurological disorders.

Congenital clubfoot (equinovarus foot, talipes equinovarus)

This is one of most common congenital conditions affecting the foot. It is more common in males, and half of the cases are bilateral. Clubfoot can be associated with other congenital abnormalities, such as developmental dysplasia of the hip, dwarfism, hand anomalies, myelomeningocele. Clubfoot is characterized by forefoot adduction, hindfoot varus, and equinus (calcaneus is inverted under the talus). It is mostly treated by sequential casting (Ponseti method).

INDEX